Keto Diet Cakes Recipes for Beginners

Boost your Metabolism and your Health with this Complete and Delicious Collection of Keto Diet

Jessica Simpson

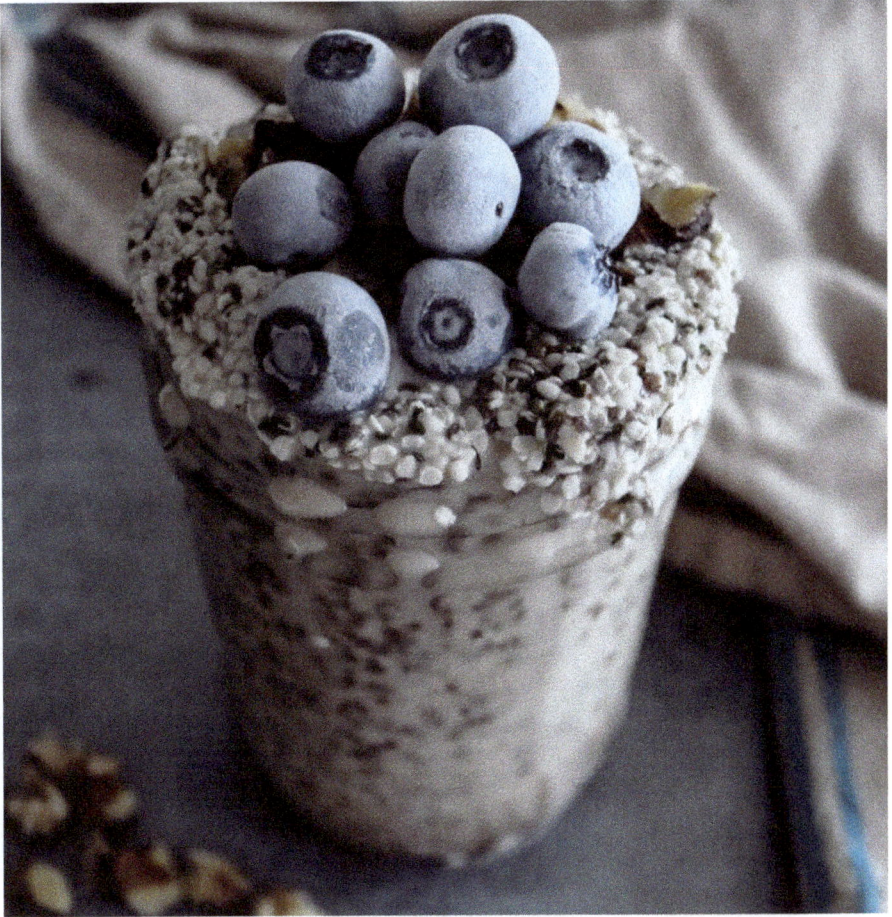

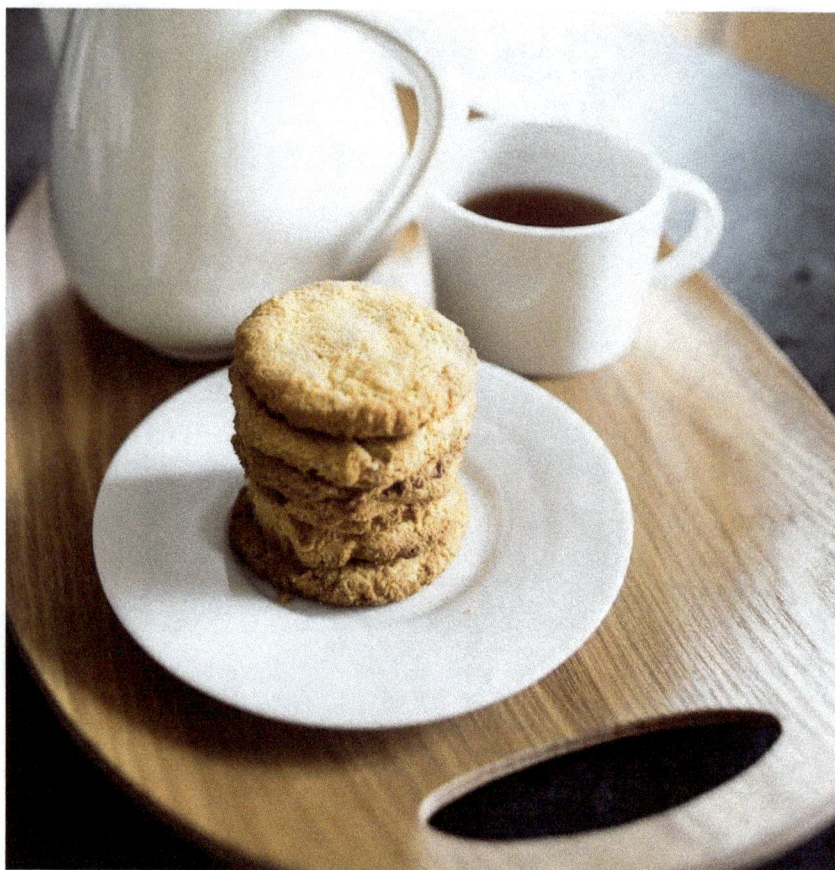

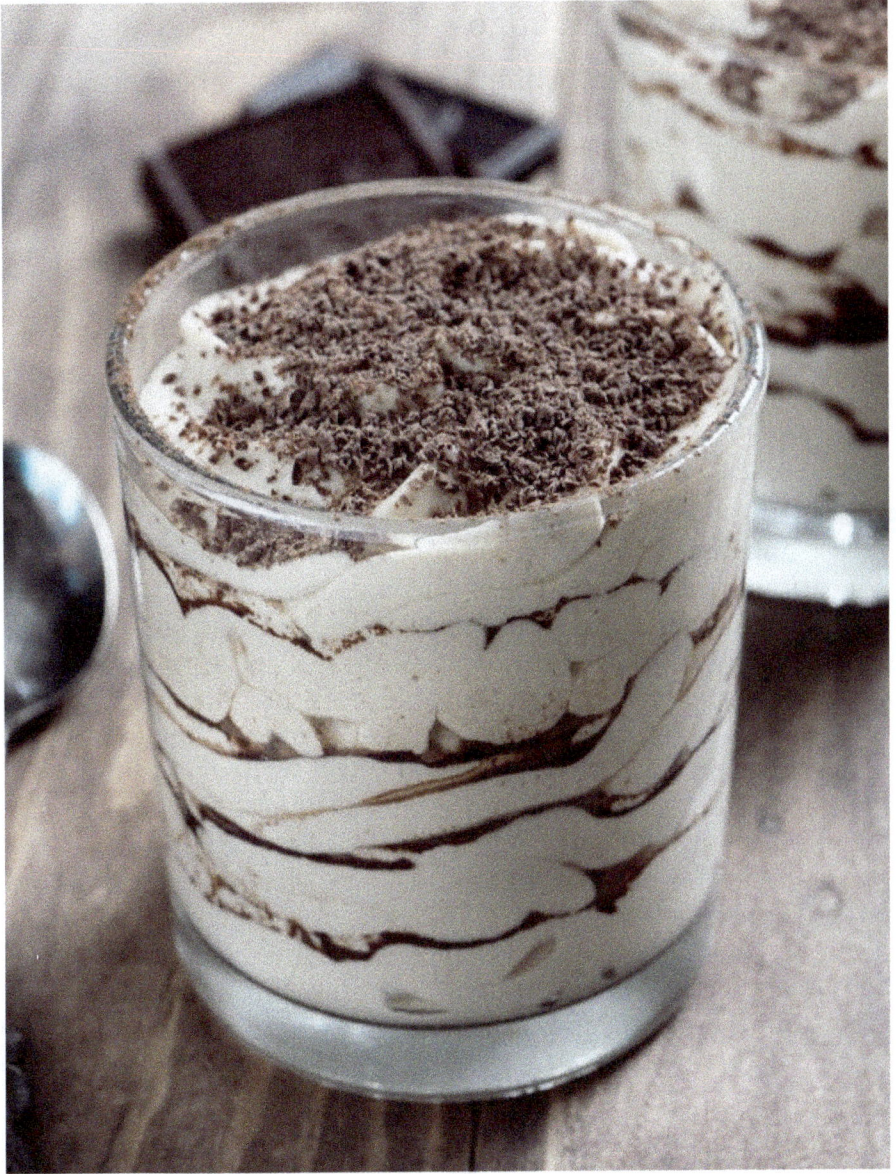

Contents

Birthday Cake

Servings: 16

Cooking Time: 1 Hour 45 Minutes + 3 Hours 40 Minutes With Sprinkles

Ingredients:

- For the cake:
- 40 drops Stevia drops, vanilla flavored
- 1/4 cup coconut flour
- 1 3/4 cup Swerve sweetener, granulated
- 1 cup almond flour
- 3 large eggs
- 1 tsp. baking powder, gluten-free
- 4 tbsp. coconut milk
- Coconut oil cooking spray
- 16 tbsp. coconut oil
- 1 tsp. vanilla extract, sugar-free
- 1 tsp. maple extract
- 1/2 tsp. salt
- For the frosting:
- 2 medium avocados, peeled
- 1/2 tsp. salt
- 2 oz. dark chocolate, unsweetened
- 3/4 cup Swerve sweetener, confectioner
- 1/2 tsp. maple extract

- 22 drops Stevia drops, vanilla flavored
- For the sprinkles: (optional)
- 3-6 drops food coloring
- 8 oz. coconut, unsweetened and shredded
- 1 tsp. water

Directions:

1. Sprinkles:
2. Make the sprinkles the day before as they need to dry overnight. Prepare a cookie sheet with a piece of wax or baking paper.
3. Place 8 tablespoons of coconut in a dish. Add 6 drops of food coloring and 1 teaspoon of water. Stir until the coloring is what you desire, adding more food coloring or water if needed.
4. Transfer to the prepared cookie sheet and put in a place it will be undisturbed overnight so the coconut can dry.
5. Repeat the steps for additional colors, if you prefer.
6. Cake:
7. Note: the recipe ingredients above is only for one layer of cake. Double the recipe if you want a two layer cake.
8. Set your stove to be at the temperature of 350° Fahrenheit. Trim a circle of baking sheet to match the size of the springform pan.Apply the cooking spray liberally inside and place the baking paper in the base

of the pan. Spray additional cooking spray on top of the baking paper.

9. In a food processor on the setting of high, beat the sweetener, coconut oil, liquid stevia, and salt together for 30 seconds.

10. Add in the maple extract to the mixture.

11. Blend the coconut milk, vanilla extract, and eggs to the bowl and pulse for 30 seconds more.

12. Pour the almond and coconut flours for an additional 30 seconds. The mixture will have the consistency of dry cake batter at this point. With a rubber scraper, carefully stir the rainbow sprinkles (optional) into the batter until incorporated.

13. Transfer the cake batter to the springform pan and heat for 35 minutes. Check with a toothpick to ensure the cake is baked fully in the middle.

14. Move the cake pan onto a cutting board. Wait for approximately 5 minutes and unlock the pan.

15. Frosting:

16. Heat a saucepan to melt the chocolate fully.Using the food processor on the high setting, pulse the avocados and sweetener until smooth.

17. Add the liquid Stevia, maple extract and salt until combined.For the desired consistency, you can add 1 teaspoon of water until the frosting thins. Be sure all

ingredients are mixed thoroughly by scraping the sides between pulses.

18. Taste test the frosting and add additional sweetener if preferred.

19. Frosting the cake:

20. Ensure that the cake(s) has cooled completely before frosting.

21. Move the cake onto the center of a cake plate.

22. Start by frosting the middle of the top and finish with the sides.If you have more than one layer, frost the middle of the first layer. Then stack the other cake above. Frost the top and then frost the sides.

23. Add more sprinkles on top of the cake, if desired and serve!

24. Tricks and Tips:

25. The recipe for the frosting will also work for icing 12 cupcakes or can be put in a container with a lid in the refrigerator when ready to use.The cake can be frozen and defrosted in the refrigerator a day before you are ready to frost.

26. The leftover sprinkles can be stored in a mason jar and placed in the pantry until the next celebration.

Nutrition Info: 6 grams ;Net Carbs: 3.2 grams ;Fat: 21 grams ;Calories: 282

Keto Celebration Brownie Cake

Servings: 25-30

Cooking Time: 22 Minutes

Ingredients:

- For cake (wet ingredients):
- 4 bars dark chocolate, stevia sweetened, break into smaller pieces
- 12 large eggs
- 3 cups powdered erythritol
- 17.5 ounces coconut oil or butter
- 60 drops liquid stevia
- For cake (dry ingredients)
- 4 cups almond flour
- 1 cup ground chia seeds
- 4 teaspoons cream of tartar
- 2 cups cacao powder or cocoa powder
- 2 teaspoons baking soda
- For filling:
- 2 ½ cups double cream
- 5 cups mixed berries
- 7 ounces full-fat Greek yogurt

Directions:

1. To make cake: Add chocolate and butter into a heatproof bowl. Place the bowl in a double boiler.

2. Stir frequently. When nearly all the chocolate is melted, turn off the heat. Let the bowl remain in the double boiler and stir until it melts completely. Remove the bowl from the double boiler and set aside to cool.

3. Add eggs, sweetener and stevia into a bowl. Beat with an electric hand mixer until well incorporated.

4. Add the cooled chocolate and beat well.

5. Add all the dry ingredients into another bowl and stir. Transfer into the bowl of wet ingredients. Fold gently.

6. Take 2 cake pans or springform pans of about 10 inches each. Grease with cooking spray. Line with parchment paper.

7. Pour 1/3 of the batter into one pan and 2/3 of the batter into another pan.

8. Bake in a preheated oven at 350° F for about 35-40 minutes. A toothpick when inserted in the center should come out clean when the cake is ready. Remove the smaller cake (with 1/3 batter) after about 22-25 minutes.

9. Remove the cake from the oven and from the pans. Cool completely on a wire rack.

10. To make filling: Add cream and yogurt into a bowl and beat with an electric hand mixer until stiff, making sure not to over beat.

11. Cut the bigger cake into 3 even sections, horizontally. So you have 3 cakes in all.

12. Place one cake on a serving platter. Spoon half the cream filling over the cake.

13. Place half the berries randomly over the filling.

14. Place the next cake over the berries. Spoon half the cream filling over the cake.

15. Place half the berries randomly over the filling.

16. Place the last cake over the berries.

17. Chill for 30 minutes.

18. Slice and serve.

19. Leftovers can be stored in an airtight container in the refrigerator. The cake can keep for 5 days.

Nutrition Info: Per Servings: Calories: 302.5 kcal, Fat: 28 g, Carbohydrates: 7.7 g, Protein: 6.3 g

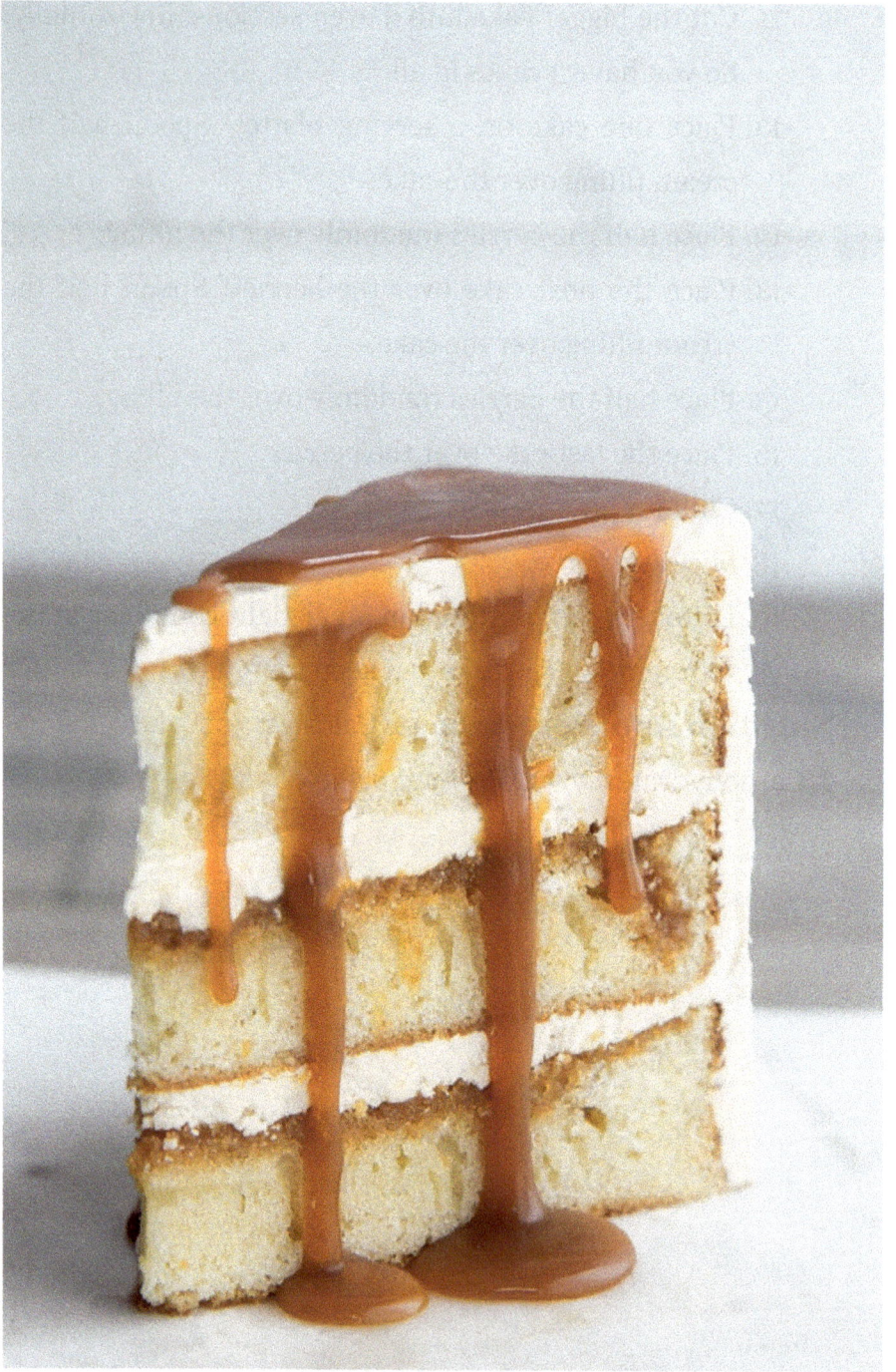

Caramel Cake

Servings: 6

Cooking Time: 30 Minutes

Ingredients:

- 2 1/2 cups almond flour
- 3/4 cup almond milk
- 1/4 cup protein powder (without flavour)
- 1 tbsp baking powder
- 1/2 cup butter, melted
- 1/4 cup coconut flour
- 2/3 cup swerve
- 4 large eggs
- 1 tsp vanilla essence
- 1/2 tsp salt
- 2 batches sugar-free caramel sauce

Directions:

1. Cake
2. Let your oven preheat at 3 degrees F. Grease 2- 8-inch baking pan with cooking oil.
3. Layer these pans with parchment paper and set them aside.
4. Mix both flours, protein, salt, and baking powder in a medium bowl.

5. Mix and beat butter with sweetener in a mixer until fluffy.

6. Whisk in all eggs one by one and vanilla.

7. Now stir in the coconut flour mix and coconut milk into the egg's mixture.

8. Divide this batter into the two pans. Bake them for 25 minutes.

9. Allow the baked cake to cool on wire rack.

10. Caramel Glaze

11. Cook the sugar-free caramel sauce in a saucepan until it bubbles.

12. Remove the glaze from the heat and allow it to cool.

13. Place on the cake over a plate and top it with 1/3 caramel sauce.

14. Spread the prepared glaze evenly and allow it to sit for 10 minutes.

15. Now place the second cake over it and pour the remaining caramel sauce on top.

16. Slice and serve.

Nutrition Info: Per Servings: Calories 264 Total Fat 23.4 g Saturated Fat 11.7 g Cholesterol 135 mg Total Carbs 2.5 g Sugar 12.5 g Fiber 1 g Sodium 112 mg Potassium 65 mg Protein 7.9 g

Vanilla Butter Cake

Servings: 9

Cooking Time: 35 Minutes

Ingredients:

- 5 eggs
- 1 tsp baking powder
- oz almond flour
- 12 cup butter, softened
- 1 cup Swerve
- 4 oz cream cheese, softened
- 1 tsp vanilla
- 1 tsp orange extract

Directions:

1. Preheat the oven to 350 F 0 C.
2. Spray 9-inch cake pan with cooking spray and set aside.
3. Add all ingredients into the mixing bowl and whisk until batter is fluffy.
4. Pour batter into the prepared pan and bake in preheated oven for 35- minutes.
5. Remove cake from oven and set aside to cool completely.
6. Slices and serve.

Nutrition Info: Per Servings: Net Carbs: 3.3g; Calories: 289; Total Fat: 22g; Saturated Fat: 10.7g Protein: 8.5g; Carbs: 5.5g; Fiber: 2.2g; Sugar: 1.1g; Fat 85% Protein 11% Carbs 4%

Italian Pecan Cake

Servings: 8

Cooking Time: 45 Minutes

Ingredients:

- Cake
- 1/2 cup butter softened
- 1 cup Swerve
- 4 large eggs, separated
- 1/2 cup heavy cream
- 1 teaspoon vanilla essence
- 1 1/2 cups almond flour
- 1/2 cup coconut, shredded
- 1/2 cup pecans, chopped
- 1/4 cup coconut flour
- 2 teaspoons baking powder
- 1/2 teaspoon salt
- 1/4 teaspoon tartar cream
- Frosting
- 8 ounces cream cheese softened
- 1/2 cup heavy whipping cream
- 1/2 cup butter softened
- 1 cup powdered Swerve
- 1 teaspoon vanilla essence
- Garnish

- 2 tablespoons coconut, shredded lightly toasted
- 2 tablespoons pecans, chopped lightly toasted

Directions:

1. Cake
2. Let your oven preheat at 3 degrees F.
3. Take two 8 inches baking pan and grease them with butter.
4. Beat egg yolks with cream, sweetener, butter, and vanilla in a mixed.
5. Combine all the flours, chopped pecans, salt, baking powder, and coconut shred.
6. Add this mixture to the egg yolk batter and mix well.
7. Beat egg whites separately in a mixer until foamy.
8. Fold this foamy mixture into the flour batter.
9. Now divide the batter into the baking pans.
10. Bake them for 45 minutes in the preheated oven.
11. Remove each cake from their baking pan and let them cool on the wire rack.
12. Frosting
13. Combine all the ingredients for frosting in a mixer until frothy.
14. Keep it aside.
15. To Assemble
16. First place one cake on a plate.
17. Spread a layer of half of the frosting over its top evenly.

18. Place the second cake over it and cover it with remaining frosting.

19. Garnish it with coconut shred and pecans.

20. Chill the cake in the refrigerator for 30 minutes or more to chill.

21. Slice and serve.

Nutrition Info: Calories 267 ;Total Fat 44.5 g ;Saturated Fat 17.4 g ;Cholesterol 153 mg ;Sodium 217 mg ;Total Carbs 8.4 g ;Sugar 2.3 g ;Fiber 1.3 g ;Protein 3.1 g

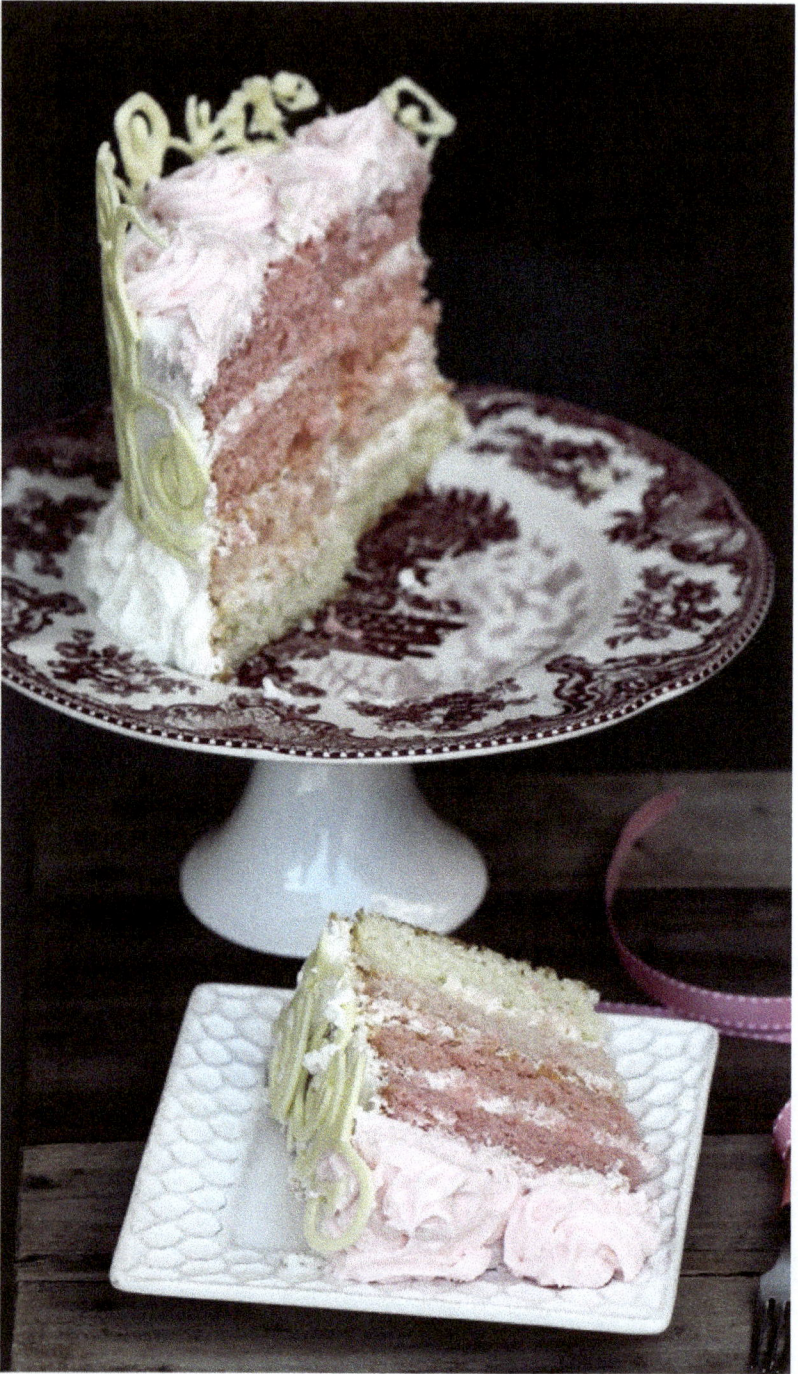

Layered Cream Cake

Servings: 8

Cooking Time: 30 Minutes

Ingredients:

- Cream Cheese Icing:
- 8 oz. cream cheese softened
- 1/2 cup butter softened
- 1/2 cup powdered Swerve
- 1 teaspoon vanilla essence optional
- 2 tablespoons heavy cream
- Carrot Cake Layers:
- 5 eggs large
- 3/4 cup erythritol
- 2 teaspoons vanilla essence
- 14 tablespoons butter melted
- 1/4 teaspoon unsweetened coconut, shredded
- 1/4 teaspoon salt
- 1/2 cup coconut flour
- 1 3/4 cup almond flour
- 2 teaspoons baking powder
- 1 1/2 teaspoon cinnamon, ground
- 1 1/4 cup shredded carrots

Directions:

1. Beat all the ingredients for icing in an electric mixer until foamy. Set it aside.
2. For carrot cake layers:
3. Preheat your oven to 0 degrees F.
4. Lay the inside of two 8 inch baking pan with parchment paper.
5. Grease the baking pans and set them aside.
6. Beat eggs with erythritol in an electric mixer for 5 minutes until foamy.
7. Mix coconut flour, salt, almond flour, baking powder, and cinnamon.
8. Transfer this mixture to the egg batter and mix well until smooth.
9. Fold in coconut, butter, melted, and carrots. Stir well.
10. Divide the cake batter into two pans and bake for 30 minutes.
11. Allow them to cook for 10 to 15 minutes.
12. To Assemble:
13. Top 1 cake with half of the icing mixture.
14. Place another cake on top of it.
15. Spread the remaining icing on the top of the upper layer.
16. Garnish as desired.
17. Slice and serve.

Nutrition Info: Calories 307 ;Total Fat 29 g ;Saturated Fat 14g ;Cholesterol 111 Mg ;Sodium 122 Mg ;Total Carbs 7 g ;Sugar 1 g ;Fiber 3 g ;Protein 6 g

Delicious Ricotta Cake

Servings: 8

Cooking Time: 45 Minutes

Ingredients:

- 2 eggs
- ½ cup erythritol
- ¼ cup coconut flour
- 15 oz ricotta
- Pinch of salt

Directions:

1. Preheat the oven to 350 F 0 C.
2. Spray 9-inch baking pan with cooking spray and set aside.
3. In a bowl whisk eggs.
4. Add remaining ingredients and mix until well combined.
5. Transfer batter in prepared baking pan.
6. Bake in preheated oven for 45 minutes.
7. Remove baking pan from oven and allow to cool completely.
8. Slice and serve.

Nutrition Info: Per Servings: Net Carbs: 2.; Calories: 91; Total Fat: 5.4g; Saturated Fat: 3g Protein: 7.5g; Carbs: 3.1g; Fiber: 0.2g; Sugar: 0.3g; Fat 55% Protein 33% Carbs 12%

Chocó Coconut Cake

Servings: 9

Cooking Time: 25 Minutes

Ingredients:

- 6 eggs
- 1 tsp vanilla
- 3 oz butter, melted
- 11.5 oz heavy whipping cream
- 2 tsp baking powder
- 3 oz unsweetened cocoa powder
- 5 oz erythritol
- 3.5 oz coconut flour

Directions:

1. Preheat the oven to 350 F 0 C.
2. In a bowl, mix together coconut flour, butter, 5.5 oz heavy whipping cream, eggs, baking powder 1.5 oz cocoa powder, and 3 oz erythritol until well combined.
3. Pour batter into the greased cake pan and bake in preheated oven for 25 minutes.
4. Remove cake from oven and allow to cool completely.
5. In a large bowl, beat remaining heavy whipping cream, cocoa powder, and erythritol until smooth.
6. Spread the cream on the cake evenly.
7. Place cake in the refrigerator for 30 minutes.

8. Slice and serve.

Nutrition Info: Per Servings: Net Carbs: 5g; Calories: 282 Total Fat: 26.1g; Saturated Fat: 15.6g Protein: 7.1g; Carbs: 10.1g; Fiber: 5.1g; Sugar: 0.; Fat 83% Protein 10% Carbs 7%

Delicious Almond Cake

Servings: 16

Cooking Time: 40 Minutes

Ingredients:

- 4 eggs
- 1 tsp baking powder
- 1 12 tsp vanilla
- 13 cup Swerve
- 2 oz cream cheese, softened
- 2 tbsp butter
- 1 cup almond flour
- 12 cup coconut flour
- 4 oz half and half
- Pinch of salt
- For topping:
- 34 cup almonds, toasted and sliced
- 13 cup Swerve
- 6 tbsp butter, melted
- 1 cup almond flour

Directions:

1. Preheat the oven to 350 F 0 C.
2. Spray 8-inch cake pan with cooking spray and set aside.

3. Add all ingredients except topping ingredients into the large bowl whisk until well combined.
4. Pour batter into the prepared cake pan and spread evenly.
5. Combine together all topping ingredients.
6. Sprinkle topping mixture evenly on top of batter.
7. Bake for 40 minutes.
8. Remove from oven and allow to cool completely.
9. Slice and serve.

Nutrition Info: Per Servings: Net Carbs: 2.8g; Calories: 198 Total Fat: 18.2g; Saturated Fat: 6g Protein: 5.9g; Carbs: 5g; Fiber: 2.2g; Sugar: 0.9g; Fat 83% Protein 12% Carbs 5%

Vanilla Cake

Servings: 12

Cooking Time: 2 Hours;

Ingredients:

- 1 1/2 cup almond flour
- 1/4 cup coconut flour
- 1 teaspoon baking powder
- 1/4 teaspoon salt
- 2 scoops Vanilla Collagen Powder
- 1 teaspoon vanilla extract, unsweetened
- 1/4 cup melted butter, unsalted
- 3 eggs
- 1/4 cup sour cream
- 1 cup almond milk

Directions:

1. Set oven to 350 degrees F and let preheat.
2. In the meantime, take an 8 by 4-inch loaf pan, grease with oil, then line with parchment paper and set aside.
3. Stir together all the dry ingredients in a large bowl until combined.
4. Crack eggs in another bowl, add vanilla and beat for 1 minute until fluffy.
5. Then beat in butter, sour cream and milk for 30 seconds until smooth.

6. Stir the mixture into flour mixture, in 2 to 3 batches, until well mixed and then let sit for 2 minutes.

7. Spoon the batter into prepared pan and bake for 50 to 60 minutes or until top is nicely golden brown and inserted toothpick into the cake comes out clean.

8. When done, let cake cool on wire rack for 15 minutes, then take it out to cool completely on wire rack and slice to serve.

Nutrition Info: Calories: 175 Cal, Carbs: 5 g, Fat: 15 g, Protein: 7 g, Fiber: 3 g.

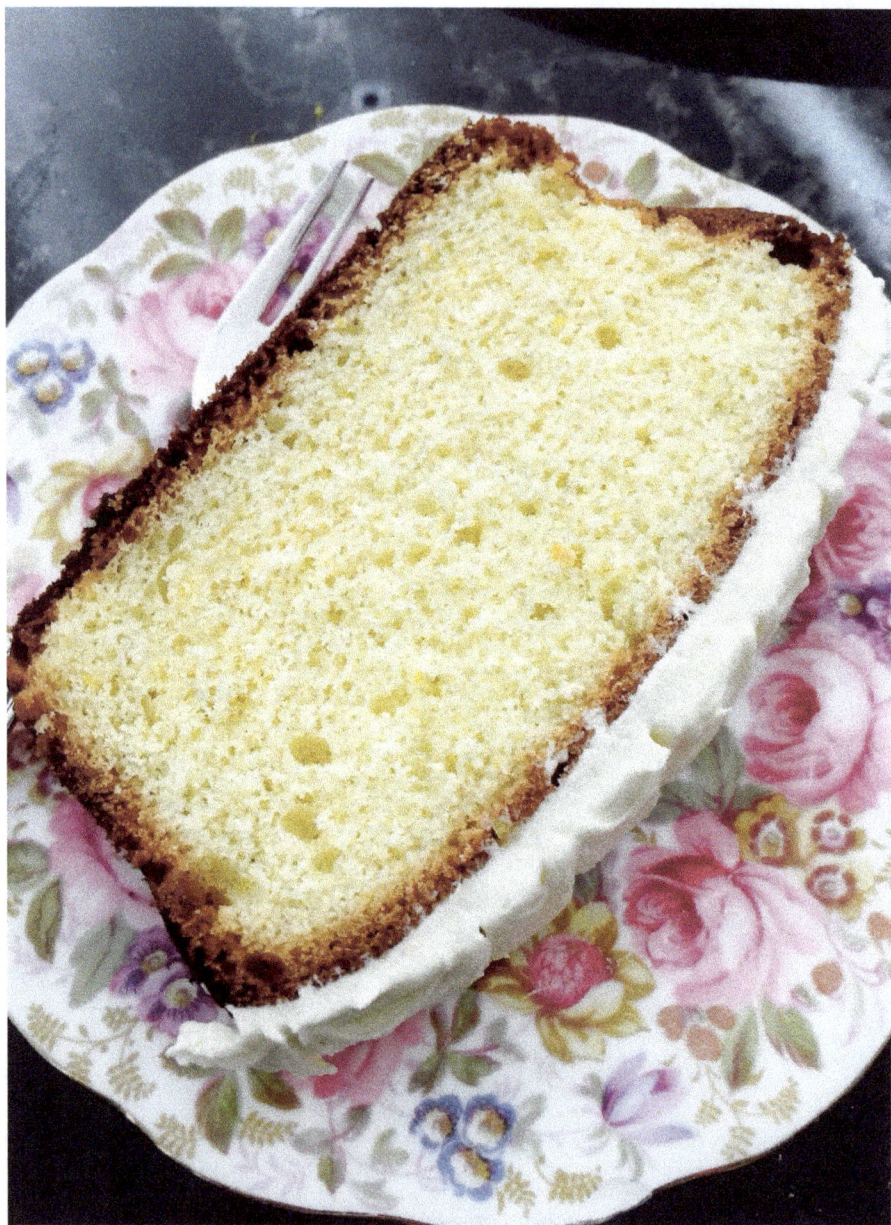

Butter Cake

Servings: 20

Cooking Time: 40 Minutes

Ingredients:

- For bottom layer:
- 6 tablespoons coconut flour
- 2 teaspoons baking powder
- 1 cup butter, at room temperature
- 4 large eggs, at room temperature
- ½ cup powdered erythritol
- 2 tablespoons gelatin (optional)
- 1 teaspoon vanilla extract
- For top layer:
- ½ cup butter, at room temperature
- ½ cup powdered erythritol
- Liquid stevia drops (80-100 drops) to taste
- 16 ounces cream cheese, at room temperature
- 1 teaspoon vanilla extract
- 4 large eggs, at room temperature

Directions:

1. Grease 2 springform pans (8 inches each) with coconut oil spray.

2. To make the bottom layer: Place butter, eggs and vanilla into a mixing bowl. Beat with an electric mixer until creamy.

3. Stir in the flour, baking powder, erythritol, gelatin and baking powder with a spatula until combined.

4. To make top layer: Add butter and cream cheese into a mixing bowl. Beat with an electric hand mixer until creamy.

5. To assemble: Divide the bottom layer among the prepared pans. Tap the pans lightly on the countertop to release any tiny air pockets.

6. Divide and spread the top layer over the bottom layer. Again, tap the pans lightly to release any tiny air pockets.

7. Bake in a preheated oven at 350° F for about 30-35 minutes. Bake in batches if necessary.

8. Remove from oven and place on a wire rack. Cool completely.

9. Slice and serve.

10. Leftovers can be stored in an airtight container in the refrigerator. The cake can keep for a week.

Nutrition Info: Per Servings: Calories: 237 kcal, Fat: 23.2 g, Carbohydrates: 2.6 g, Protein: 4.2 g

Lemon Coconut Cake

Servings: 6

Cooking Time: 45 Minutes

Ingredients:

- Coconut Cake
- 1/2 cup coconut flour
- 5 eggs
- 1/4 cup erythritol
- 1/2 cup butter melted
- 1/2 lemon juiced
- 1/2 tsp lemon zest
- 1/2 tsp xanthan gum
- 1/2 tsp salt
- Icing
- 1 cup cream cheese
- 3 tbsp powdered erythritol
- 1 tsp vanilla essence
- 1/2 tsp lemon zest

Directions:

1. Separate egg yolks from egg whites.
2. Beat the egg whites in an electric mixer until peaks are formed.
3. Add the remaining ingredients in the egg yolk bowl.

4. Fold in the egg whites gently and mix until well incorporated.

5. Spread this batter in a greased loaf pan of 9xinches.

6. Bake it for 45 minutes at 335 degrees F.

7. Meanwhile, beat all the ingredients for cream cheese frosting in the electric mixer.

8. Once the cake is baked, allow it cool on wire rack.

9. Spread the frosting over the cake.

10. Refrigerate for 4 hours then slice to serve.

Nutrition Info: Per Servings: Calories 173 Total Fat 16.2 g Saturated Fat 9.8 g Cholesterol 100 mg Total Carbs 9.4 g Sugar 0.2 g Fibre1 g Sodium 42 mg Potassium 43 mg Protein 3.3 g

Lemon Custard Cake

Servings: 8

Cooking Time: 70 Minutes

Ingredients:

- 5 eggs, room temperature, whites separated from yolks
- 1 teaspoon vanilla essence
- 2/3 cup powdered erythritol
- 1/2 cup butter, unsalted, melted
- 1 cup superfine blanched almond flour
- 1/4 cup coconut flour
- 1 3/4 cup almond milk
- 1/4 cup lemon juice
- 2 tablespoons grated lemon zest

Directions:

1. Let your oven preheat at 325 degrees F.
2. Layer an 8-inch baking dish with parchment paper.
3. Beat all the egg whites in an electric mixer until fluffy and set it aside.
4. Whisk egg yolks with sweeteners with a mixer until pale in color.
5. Stir in vanilla and melted butter.
6. Beat the mixture until smooth.

7. Add both flours, lemon zest, and juice, almond milk while beating the mixture slowly.
8. Finally, fold in the egg whites and mix gently.
9. Spread this batter in the baking dish and bake it for 70 minutes.
10. Allow the cake to cool then refrigerate for 2 hours.
11. Garnish with powder erythritol.
12. Slice and serve.

Nutrition Info: Per Servings: Calories 267 Total Fat 44.5 g Saturated Fat 17.4 g Cholesterol 153 mg Total Carbs 8.4 g Sugar 2.3 g Fiber 1.3 g Sodium 217 mg Potassium 101 mg Protein 3.1 g

Chunky Carrot Cake

Servings: 8

Cooking Time: 30 Minutes

Ingredients:

- 3/4 cup erythritol
- 3/4 cup butter
- 1 teaspoon vanilla essence
- 1/2 teaspoon pineapple extract
- 4 large egg
- 2 1/2 cup almond flour
- 2 teaspoons gluten-free baking powder
- 2 teaspoons cinnamon
- 1/2 teaspoon sea salt
- 2 1/2 cup carrots, grated
- 1 cup pecans, chopped
- Pecans, to garnish

Directions:

1. Let your oven preheat at 350 degrees F.
2. Grease the base of two 9 inch baking dishes and layer it with parchment paper.
3. Beat erythritol in cream in a suitable bowl.
4. Stir in vanilla essence and pineapple extract.
5. While beating this mixture start adding eggs one by one.

6. Add cinnamon, salt, baking powder and flour in this mixture.

7. Whisk well to combine.

8. Fold in 1 cup chopped pecans and carrots.

9. Divide the entire batter in the two pans.

10. Bake them for 30 minutes in the preheated oven.

11. Remove both the cakes from the pans and let them cool for 10 minutes on wire racks.

12. Use the remaining pecans to garnish it.

13. Slice and serve.

Nutrition Info: Calories 359 ;Total Fat 34 g ;Saturated Fat 10.3 g ;Cholesterol 112 mg ;Sodium 92 mg ;Total Carbs 8.5 g ;Sugar 2 g ;Fiber 1.3 g ;Protein 7.5 g

Lemon Pound Cake

Servings: 16

Cooking Time: 1 Hour 25 Minutes

Ingredients:

- For the cake:
- 2 1/2 cups almond flour
- 1 tsp. lemon extract
- 8 oz. cream cheese
- 1 1/2 cups Swerve sweetener, confectioner
- 4 oz. butter
- 1 1/2 tsp. baking powder, gluten-free

- 8 large eggs
- 1 1/2 tsp. vanilla extract, sugar-free
- 1/2 tsp. salt
- For the topping:
- 1/4 cup Swerve sweetener, confectioner
- 3 tbsp. heavy whipping cream
- 1/2 tsp. vanilla extract, sugar-free

Directions:

1. In a regular dish, combine sweetener with butter with an electrical beater until smooth. Add the cream cheese, baking powder and vanilla extract and continue to blend the mixture together.
2. Combine the eggs and lemon extract until the batter is incorporated.
3. Blend in the almond flour and salt, making sure no lumps are left in the batter.
4. Set your stove to the temperature of 350° Fahrenheit. Use butter to grease a regular sized cake pan.Distribute the batter in the prepared cake pan and heat in the stove for 60 minutes. Stick a toothpick into the middle to ensure it is thoroughly baked.
5. While the cake is in the stove, use a regular dish to blend the sweetener, vanilla extract, and heavy whipping cream and use an electrical beater to combine until creamy.

6. Remove the cake pan to the counter for 30 minutes to cool before putting the frosting on top.

Nutrition Info: grams ;Net Carbs: 3.4 grams ;Fat: 22 grams ;Calories: 255

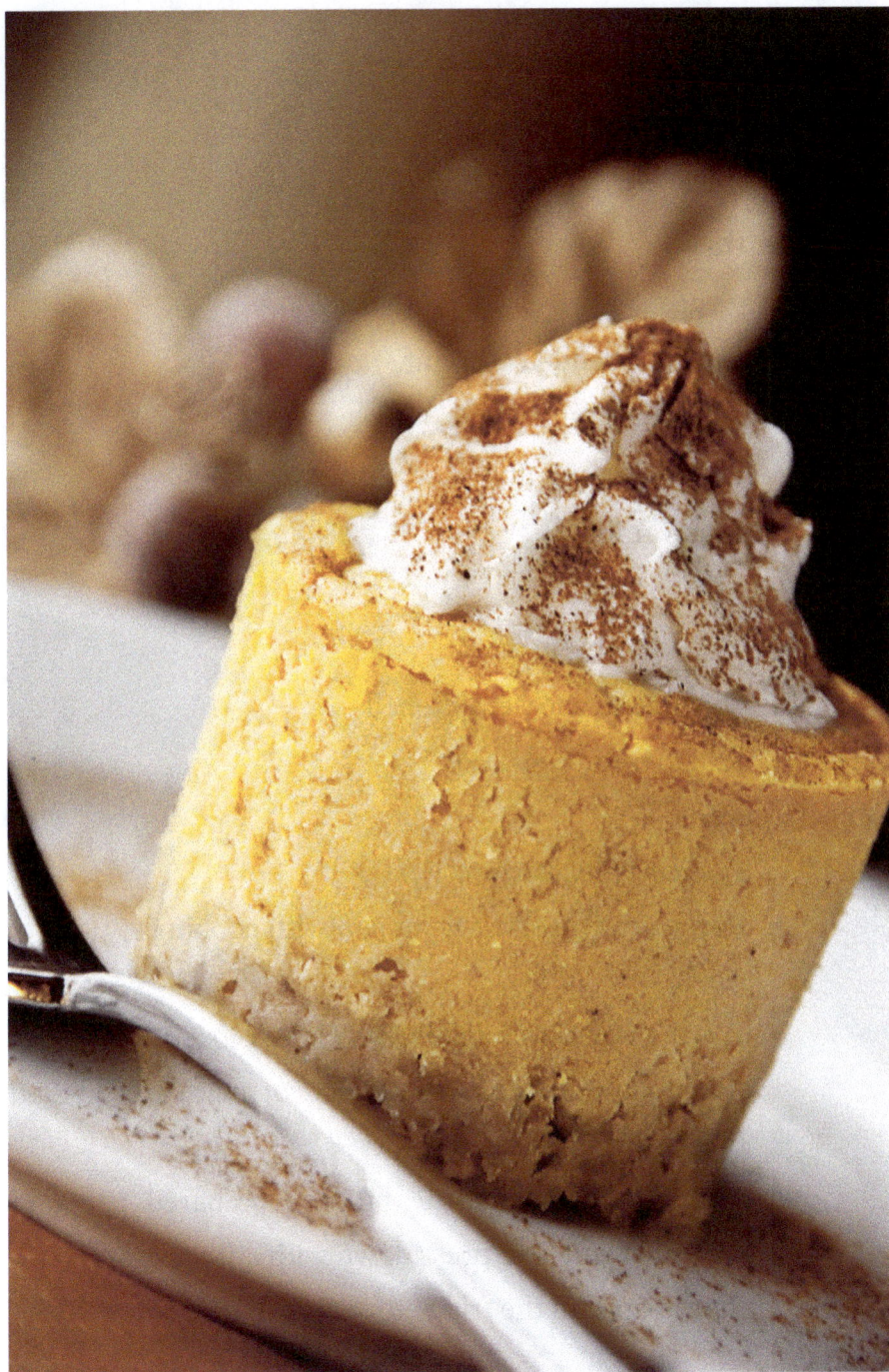

Delicious Cheesecake

Servings: 8

Cooking Time: 1 Hour 20 Minutes

Ingredients:

- 3 eggs
- 14 cup shredded coconut
- 12 cup coconut flour
- 12 cup almond flour
- 1 tsp vanilla
- 1 tbsp stevia
- 15.5 oz sour cream
- 8 oz cream cheese, softened
- 12 cup butter, melted

Directions:

1. Preheat the oven 300 F 0 C.
2. Spray 9-inch spring-form pan with cooking spray. Set aside.
3. For the crust: In a mixing bowl, mix together coconut flour, almond flour, shredded coconut, and melted butter until well combined.
4. Transfer crust mixture into the prepared pan and spread evenly and press down with a fingertip.
5. Place pan into the fridge to set crust.

6. For the cheesecake filling: In a large bowl, beat sour cream and cream cheese together.

7. Add egg, vanilla, and sweetener and beat until well combined.

8. Pour cheesecake filling evenly over crust.

9. Place pan in a water bath and bake for 1 hour-1 hour 20 minutes.

10. Remove cake pan from oven and set aside to cool completely.

11. Place cake pan into the fridge for 5-6 hours.

12. Slice and serve.

Nutrition Info: Per Servings: Net Carbs: 5.9g; Calories: 400; Total Fat: 39g; Saturated Fat: 22.3g Protein: 7.8g; Carbs: 7.2g; Fiber: 1.3g; Sugar: 2.3g; Fat 86% Protein 8% Carbs 6%

Pound Cake

Servings: 16

Cooking Time: 2 Hours And 15 Minutes

Ingredients:

- 2 ½ cups almond flour
- 1 ½ teaspoons baking powder
- ½ teaspoon salt
- 1 ½ cups erythritol sweetener
- 1 ½ teaspoons vanilla extract, unsweetened
- ½ teaspoon lemon extract, unsweetened
- ½ cup unsalted butter, softened
- 8 eggs
- 8 ounces cream cheese, chopped

Directions:

1. Set oven to 350 degrees F and let preheat.
2. In the meantime, place sweetener and butter in a bowl and beat with an electric mixer until creamy and smooth.
3. Add cream cheese and continue blending until smooth.
4. Beat in extracts and eggs, one at a time, until incorporated.
5. Stir together flour, salt, and baking powder and beat in egg mixture, ¼ cup at a time, until very smooth.

6. Spoon the batter into greased loaf pan and place into the oven to bake for 1 to 2 hours or until inserted skewer into the center of the cake comes out clean. When done, cool cake on wire rack completely and slice to serve.

Nutrition Info: Calories: 254 Cal, Carbs: 4.4 g, Fat: 23.4 g, Protein: 9 g, Fiber: 1.9 g.

Carrot Cake

Servings: 16

Cooking Time: 35 Minutes

Ingredients:

- 2 eggs
- ½ tsp vanilla
- 2 tbsp butter, melted
- ½ cup carrots, grated
- 18 tsp ground cloves
- 1 tsp cinnamon
- 1 tsp baking powder
- 2 tbsp unsweetened shredded coconut
- ¼ cup pecans, chopped
- 6 tbsp erythritol
- ¾ cup almond flour
- Pinch of salt

Directions:

1. Preheat the oven to 325 F 2 C.
2. Spray cake pan with cooking spray and set aside.
3. In a large bowl, whisk together almond flour, cloves, cinnamon, baking powder, shredded coconut, nuts, sweetener, and salt.
4. Stir in eggs, vanilla, butter, and shredded coconut until well combined.

5. Pour batter into the prepared cake pan and bake in preheated oven for 30-3minutes.

6. Slice and serve.

Nutrition Info: Per Servings: Net Carbs: 1.4g; Calories: 111 Total Fat: 10.6g; Saturated Fat: 2.2g Protein: 2.; Carbs: 3g; Fiber: 1.6g; Sugar: 0.7g; Fat 86% Protein 9% Carbs 5%

Lemon Cake

Servings: 10

Cooking Time: 60 Minutes

Ingredients:

- 4 eggs
- 2 tbsp lemon zest
- ½ cup fresh lemon juice
- ¼ cup erythritol
- 1 tbsp vanilla
- ½ cup butter softened
- 2 tsp baking powder
- ¼ cup coconut flour
- 2 cups almond flour

Directions:

1. Preheat the oven to 300 F 0 C.
2. Grease 9-inch loaf pan with butter and set aside.
3. In a large bowl, whisk all ingredients until a smooth batter is formed.
4. Pour batter into the loaf pan and bake in preheated oven for 60 minutes.
5. Slice and serve.

Nutrition Info: Per Servings: Net Carbs: 3.; Calories: 244; Total Fat: 22.3g; Saturated Fat: 7.3g Protein: 7.3g; Carbs: 6.3g; Fiber: 2.7g; Sugar: 1.5g; Fat 83% Protein 12% Carbs 5%

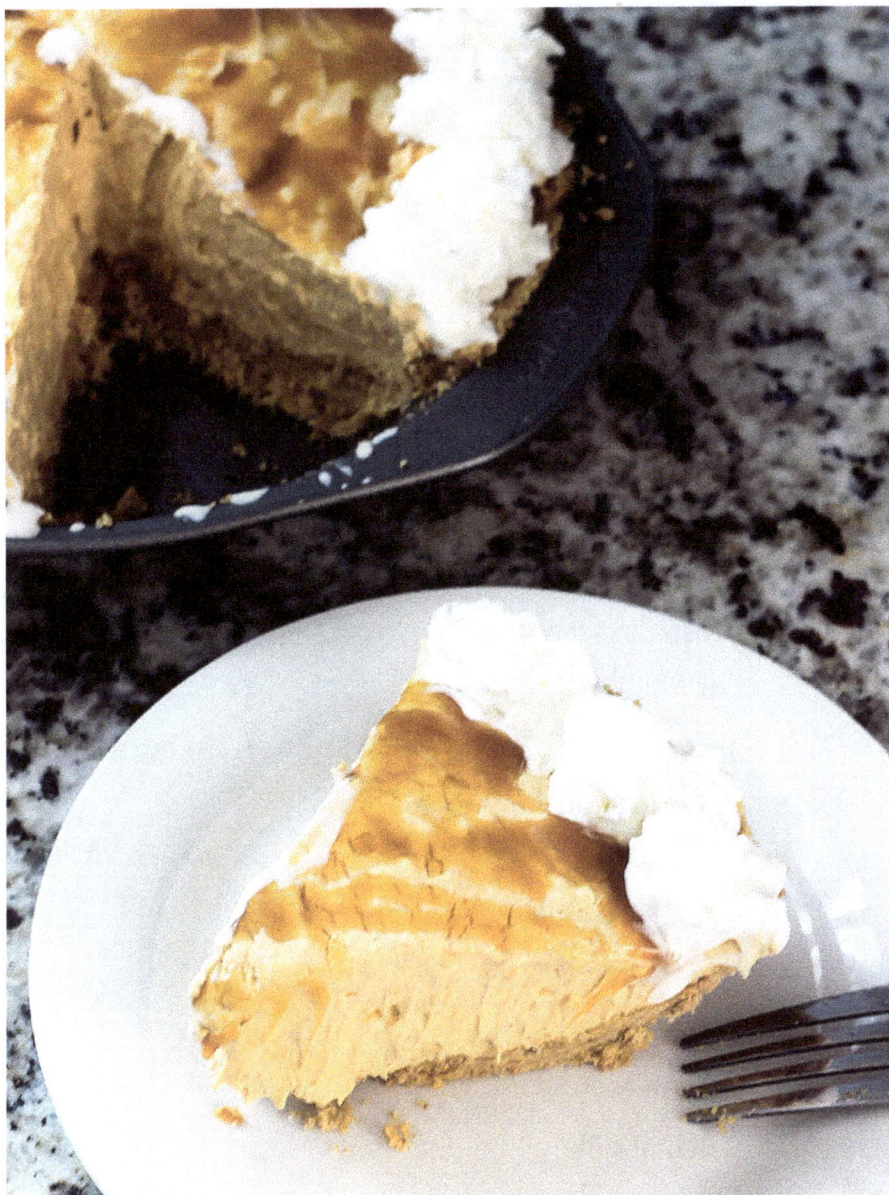

Pumpkin Cheesecake

Servings: 8

Cooking Time: 1 Hour 10 Minutes

Ingredients:

- For Crust:
- 12 cup almond flour
- 1 tbsp swerve
- 14 cup butter, melted
- 1 tbsp flaxseed meal
- For Filling:
- 3 eggs
- 12 tsp ground cinnamon
- 12 tsp vanilla
- 23 cup pumpkin puree
- 15.5 oz cream cheese
- 14 tsp ground nutmeg
- 23 cup Swerve
- Pinch of salt

Directions:

1. Preheat the oven to 300 F 0 C.
2. Spray 9-inch spring-form pan with cooking spray. Set aside.

3. For Crust: In a bowl, mix together almond flour, swerve, flaxseed meal, and salt.

4. Add melted butter and mix well to combine.

5. Transfer crust mixture into the prepared pan and press down evenly with a fingertip.

6. Bake for 10-15 minutes.

7. Remove from oven and allow to cool for 10 minutes.

8. For the cheesecake filling: In a large bowl, beat cream cheese until smooth and creamy.

9. Add eggs, vanilla, swerve, pumpkin puree, nutmeg, cinnamon, and salt and stir until well combined.

10. Pour cheesecake batter into the prepared crust and spread evenly.

11. Bake for 50-55 minutes.

12. Remove cheesecake from oven and set aside to cool completely.

13. Place cheesecake in the fridge for 4 hours.

14. Slices and serve.

Nutrition Info: Per Servings: Net Carbs: 3.9g; Calories: 320 Total Fat: 30.4g; Saturated Fat: 16.6g Protein: 8.2g; Carbs: 5.6g; Fiber: 1.7g; Sugar: 1.2g; Fat 86% Protein 10% Carbs 4%

Cheesecake

Servings: 12

Cooking Time: 5 Hours And 30 Minutes

Ingredients:

- For the Crust:
- 1 1/2 cups almond flour
- 1/4 cup monk fruit sweetener
- 4 tablespoons unsalted butter
- For the Filling:
- 1 cup monk fruit sweetener
- 3/4 teaspoon vanilla extract, unsweetened
- 3 eggs
- 24-ounce cream cheese, softened
- 1/4 cup heavy whipping cream

Directions:

1. Set oven to 350 degrees F and let preheat.
2. In the meantime, place butter in a heatproof bowl and microwave for 30 seconds or until melted.
3. Add remaining ingredients for the crust into melted butter, stir well until combined and add the mixture into 9-inch springform pan.
4. Press and spread the mixture evenly into the bottom of the pan, then place into the oven and bake for 8 minutes or until crust is nicely golden brown.

5. When done, remove crust from the oven and let cool on wire rack for 10 minutes, lower oven temperature to 32degrees F.
6. Place all the ingredients for filling in another bowl and beat using a stand mixer until well combined.
7. Spoon this mixture into cooled crust, smooth the top with a spatula and place the pan into the oven.
8. Bake cake for 1 hour and 10 minutes or until set and inserted skewer into the center of the cake comes out clean.
9. Then cover the cheesecake with aluminum foil and chill in the refrigerator for 4 hours.
10. Slice and serve.

Nutrition Info: Calories: 517 Cal, Carbs: 28.8 g, Fat: 49 g, Protein: 12.2 g, Fiber: 21.3 g.

Keto Butter Cake

Servings: 8

Cooking Time: 35 Minutes

Ingredients:

- 3 tbsp coconut flour
- 1/4 cup powdered erythritol
- 1 tsp baking powder
- 1 tbsp gelatine
- 8 tbsp butter, room temperature
- 1/2 tsp vanilla essence
- 2 large eggs, room temperature
- Top Layer
- 8 tbsp butter, room temperature
- 8 oz cream cheese, room temperature
- 1/4 cup powdered erythritol
- 1/2 tsp vanilla essence
- 50 drops liquid stevia
- 2 large eggs, room temperature

Directions:

1. Let your oven preheat at 350 degrees F.
2. Grease an 8-inch baking pan with coconut oil.
3. Bottom Layer
4. Whisk eggs with butter, vanilla essence in an electric mixer.

5. Stir in erythritol, coconut flour, baking, and gelatin.

6. Mix well and set this batter aside.

7. Top Layer

8. Beat butter with cream cheese in another bowl using a hand mixer.

9. Whisk in eggs, vanilla essence, stevia, and erythritol.

10. Mix well and set this batter aside.

11. Cake

12. Add the bottom layer batter to the prepared pan.

13. Pour the top layer batter over it and spread it evenly.

14. Bake the cake for 35 minutes in the preheated oven.

15. Allow the cake to cool at room temperature.

16. Slice and serve.

Nutrition Info: Per Servings: Calories 251 Total Fat 24.5 g Saturated Fat 14.7 g Cholesterol 165 mg Total Carbs 4.3 g Sugar 0.5 g Fiber 1 g Sodium 142 mg Potassium 80 mg Protein 5.9 g

Chocolate Buttercream Cake

Servings: 12

Cooking Time: 35 Minutes

Ingredients:

- For wet ingredients:
- 8 ounces stevia sweetened dark chocolate, chopped
- 4 large eggs
- ½ cup coconut cream
- 60 drops liquid stevia
- For dry ingredients:
- 4 tablespoons cacao powder
- 4 teaspoons baking soda
- 1 cup almond flour
- ½ teaspoon fine sea salt
- For buttercream frosting:
- 1 pound butter, softened
- Chocolate chips or cacao nibs to garnish
- 6 scoops Perfect Keto vanilla collagen MCT powder or other MCT powder

Directions:

1. Add chocolate chips into a microwave safe bowl. Microwave on high for 30-40 seconds or until melted. Whisk every -15 seconds.

2. Add coconut cream and whisk well. If the mixture is very thick, place it back in the microwave and cook for 10 seconds.

3. Keep whisking until the mixture is shiny.

4. Add eggs and stevia and whisk well.

5. Add all the dry ingredients into another bowl and stir.

6. Add into the bowl of wet ingredients and fold until just combined.

7. Grease a baking dish of about 9 x 13 inches with cooking spray. Line with parchment paper.

8. Pour the batter into the dish.

9. Bake in a preheated oven at 350° F for about 35 minutes or a toothpick when inserted in the center comes out clean. Remove from the oven and set aside to cool for a while.

10. Meanwhile make the buttercream frosting as follows: Add butter into a mixing bowl. Add MCT powder and whip with an electric mixer until creamy.

11. Cut the cake into 2 halves horizontally.

12. Spread frosting on one half of the cake. Place the other half of the cake over the frosting.

13. Spread a thin layer of frosting on top. Freeze until firm.

14. Remove from the freezer and spread the remaining frosting over the cake.

15. Scatter cocoa nibs all over the cake. Chill for 10 minutes.

16. Cut into slices and serve.

17. Leftovers can be stored in an airtight container in the refrigerator. This can keep for a week.

Nutrition Info: Per Servings: Calories: 416.2 kcal, Fat: 41.1 g, Carbohydrates: 3.7 g, Protein: 9.7 g

Vanilla Birthday Cake With Thick Vanilla Frosting

Servings: 12

Cooking Time:50 Minutes

Ingredients:

- 3 cups ground almonds
- ½ cup ground hazelnuts
- 2 tsp baking powder
- Pinch of salt
- 1 ½ tsp Stevia/your preferred keto sweetener
- 2 Tbsp vanilla extract
- 1 cup full fat sour cream
- 4 eggs
- Frosting:
- 5 oz butter, softened
- 1 lb full fat cream cheese
- 1 tsp Stevia/your preferred keto sweetener
- 2 Tbsp vanilla extract

Directions:

1. Preheat the oven to 360 degrees Fahrenheit and line a cake pan with baking paper
2. Combine the ground almonds, ground hazelnuts, baking powder, sweetener and salt in a large bowl

3. In a separate bowl, whisk together the vanilla, sour cream and eggs until combined

4. Pour the wet ingredients into the dry ingredients and stir to combine

5. Pour the batter into your prepared cake pan and place it into the oven for about 30 minutes or until the cake is lightly golden on top and bounces back when you gently press it

6. Leave the cake to cool completely before frosting

7. Make the frosting as the cake cools: beat together the butter, cream cheese, sweetener and vanilla extract until smooth and creamy

8. Slice the cake in half (so you have a top and a bottom like a sandwich)

9. Spread 1 third of the frosting onto the bottom half of the cake then place the top half of the cake on top. Spread the remaining 2 thirds of the frosting over the cake and down the sides

10. Slice, serve and enjoy!

Nutrition Info: Calories: 452;Fat: 39 grams ;Protein: grams ;Total carbs: 8 grams ;Net carbs: 5 grams

Citrus Cake with Cream Cheese Frosting

Servings: 10

Cooking Time:1 Hour

Ingredients:

- 2 cups ground almonds
- 1 tsp baking powder
- 1 tsp Stevia/your preferred keto sweetener
- 3 eggs
- 1 cup full fat sour cream
- ½ cup grapeseed oil (or any other flavorless/mild oil)
- Zest and juice of 1 lime
- Zest and juice of 1 lemon
- Zest and juice of 1 orange
- Frosting:
- 9 oz full fat cream cheese
- 4 oz butter, softened
- 1 tsp Stevia/your preferred keto sweetener
- Zest of 1 lime
- Zest of 1 lemon
- Zest of 1 orange

Directions:

1. Preheat the oven to 360 degrees Fahrenheit and line a cake pan with baking paper

69

2. In a large bowl, toss together the ground almonds, baking powder and sweetener

3. In a smaller bowl, whisk together the eggs, sour cream, oil, zest and juice of the lime, lemon and orange until combined and smooth

4. Pour the wet ingredients into the dry ingredients and stir together until combined and smooth

5. Pour the batter into your prepared cake pan and pop into your preheated oven to bake for about 40 minutes or until a skewer comes out clean

6. As the cake cools, make the frosting: beat together the cream cheese, butter, sweetener and all citrus zests until super smooth and fluffy

7. Leave the cake to cool completely before frosting with your citrus cream cheese frosting

8. Serve!

Nutrition Info: Calories: 453;Fat: 44 grams ;Protein: 8 grams ;Total carbs: 8 grams ;Net carbs: 5 grams

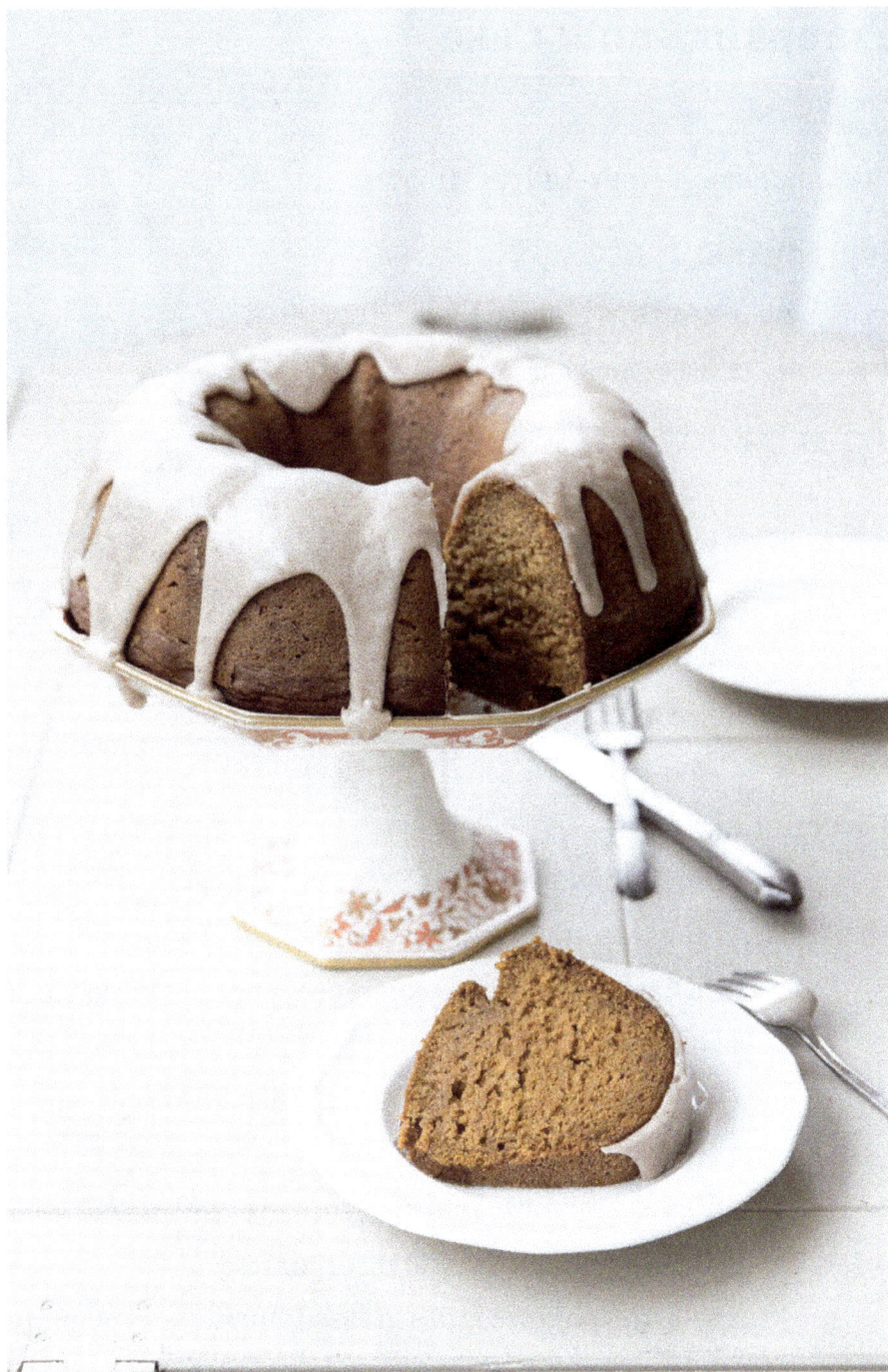

Pumpkin Bundt Cake

Servings: 12

Cooking Time: 1 Hour And 30 Minutes

Ingredients:

- 2 3/4 cups almond flour
- 2 teaspoons baking powder
- 1/2 teaspoons salt
- 1 1/3 cups Erythritol sweetener
- 2 teaspoons pumpkin pie spice
- 2 teaspoons vanilla extract, unsweetened
- 1/2 cup unsalted butter, melted
- 8.5-ounce pumpkin puree
- 6 eggs

Directions:

1. Set oven to 325 degrees F and let preheat.
2. In the meantime, stir together all the dry ingredients in a large bowl until combined and set aside until required.
3. Place all the ingredients in another bowl and whisk until smooth.
4. Add this mixture into dry mixture and whisk well using a stand mixer until incorporated.
5. Spoon the mixture into a greased Bundt pan and place into the oven to bake for 60 minutes or more until top

is nicely brown and inserted toothpick into the cake comes out clean.

6. When done, cool cake on wire rack for 15 minutes and then take out to cool completely.

7. Slice to serve.

Nutrition Info: Calories: 2 Cal, Carbs: 8 g, Fat: 26 g, Protein: 8.4 g, Fiber: 3.2 g.

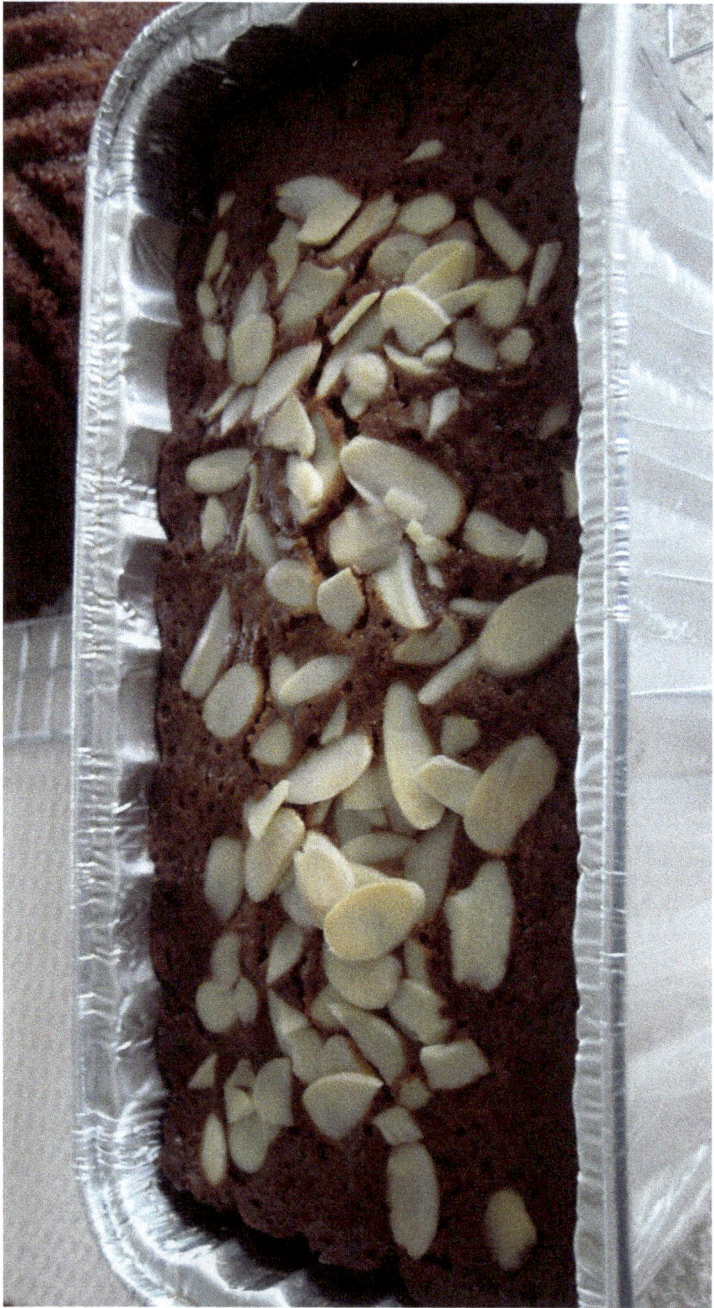

Allspice Almond Cake

Servings: 8

Cooking Time: 25 Minutes

Ingredients:

- For the cake:
- 1/2 cup erythritol
- 5 tablespoons butter softened
- 4 large eggs
- 2 tablespoons unsweetened almond milk
- 1 teaspoon vanilla
- 1 1/2 cups Almond Flour
- 2 tablespoons coconut flour
- 1 tablespoon baking powder
- 1 1/2 teaspoon cinnamon, ground
- 1/4 teaspoon ground allspice
- 1/2 cup almonds
- Cream Cheese Frosting:
- 4 oz. cream cheese softened
- 2 tablespoons butter softened
- 1 teaspoon vanilla
- 1 tablespoon heavy cream
- 1/4 cup confectioners erythritol

Directions:

1. Let your oven preheat at 350 degrees F.

2. Take a 9-inch pan and line it with a parchment paper.

3. Beat erythritol in butter in a suitable bowl until foamy.

4. Whisk in vanilla, eggs, and milk.

5. Beat well then stir in spices, coconut flour, almond flour, and baking powder.

6. Now add the almond to this batter and mix gently.

7. Pour the almond batter in the baking pan and spread it evenly.

8. Bake it for 25 minutes in the preheated oven.

9. Meanwhile, beat frosting ingredients in a bowl until creamy.

10. Once the cake is made, remove it from the pan and place it over a wire rack.

11. After ten minutes, spread the frosting over the cake evenly.

12. Refrigerate for 30 minutes or more.

13. Slice and serve.

Nutrition Info: Calories 331 ;Total Fat 38.5 g ;Saturated Fat 19.2 g ;Cholesterol mg ;Sodium 283 mg ;Total Carbs 9.2 g ;Sugar 3 g ;Fiber 1 g ;Protein 2.1 g

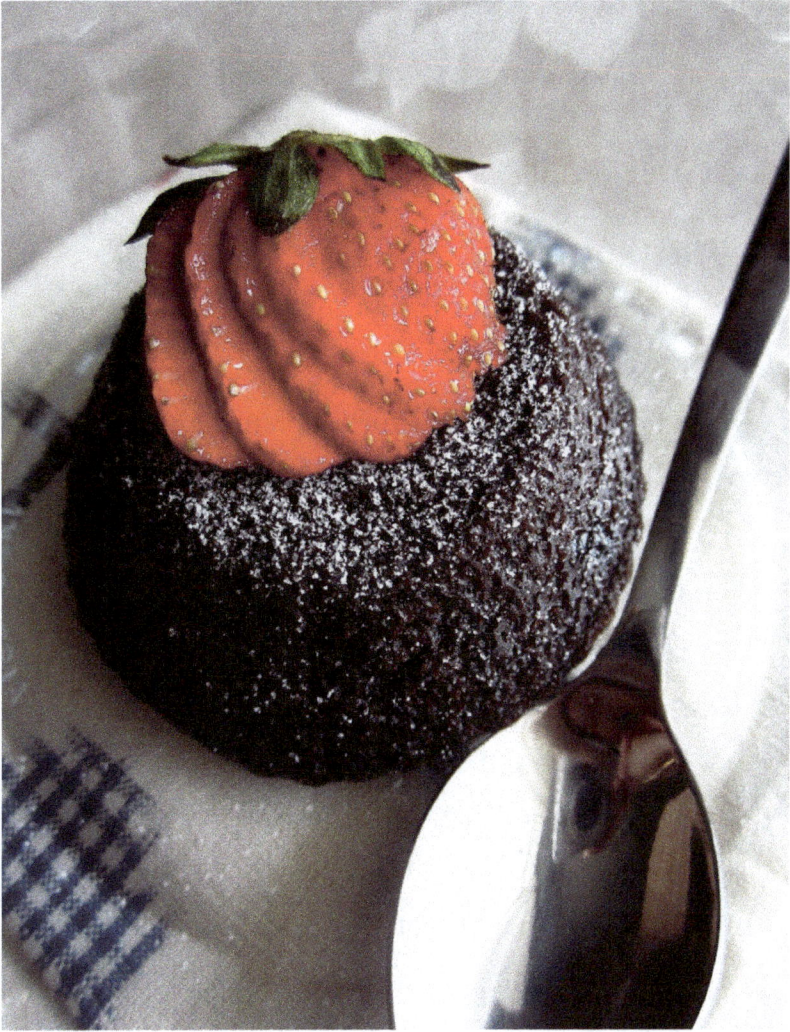

Lava Cake

Servings: 1

Cooking Time: 30 Minutes

Ingredients:

- 2 tablespoons cocoa powder, unsweetened
- 1/16 teaspoon salt
- 2 tablespoons erythritol sweetener
- 1/4 teaspoon baking powder
- 1/2 teaspoon vanilla extract, unsweetened
- 1 egg
- 1 tablespoon heavy cream

Directions:

1. Set oven to 350 degrees F and let preheat.
2. In the meantime, stir together cocoa powder and sweetener in a bowl until mixed.
3. Crack eggs in another bowl and beat until fluffy.
4. Add salt, baking powder, vanilla, eggs, and cream into cocoa mixture and stir well until incorporated.
5. Take a heatproof mug, grease with oil, then pour in prepared batter and bake for 10 to 1minutes or until cake is set.
6. Cover the mug with a plate, hold it tightly and flip it upside down multiple times to slide cake to the plate.
7. Serve straightaway.

Nutrition Info: Calories: 173 Cal, Carbs: 4 g, Fat: 13 g, Protein: g, Fiber: 2 g.

Buttery Chocolate Cake

Servings: 6

Cooking Time: 46 Minutes

Ingredients:

- 7 oz. sugar-free dark chocolate
- 3.5 oz. butter
- 3.4 oz. cream
- 4 egg whites
- 4 egg yolks
- erythritol to taste

Directions:

1. Take an 8-inch baking pan and rub some butter in it to grease it.
2. Melt the remaining butter with chocolate in the microwave then mix well.
3. Once melted add cream and erythritol to the chocolate mixture.
4. Beat in egg yolks and beat until it is well incorporated.
5. Whisk egg white within another mixing bowl until it turns foamy.
6. Fold the egg white foam into the creamy butter mixture.
7. Use a spatula to transfer the batter to the prepared baking pan.

8. Bake it in the preheated oven for 45 minutes at 325 degrees F.

9. Remove the cake from the pan and place it over the wire rack.

10. Let it cool for 5 mins then refrigerate it for 4 hours packed in a plastic sheet.

11. Slice and serve the cake.

Nutrition Info: Calories 173 ;Total Fat 16.2 g ;Saturated Fat 9.8 g ;Cholesterol 100 mg ;Sodium 42 mg ;Total Carbs 9.4 g ;Sugar 0.2 g ;Fibre1 g ;Protein 3.3 g

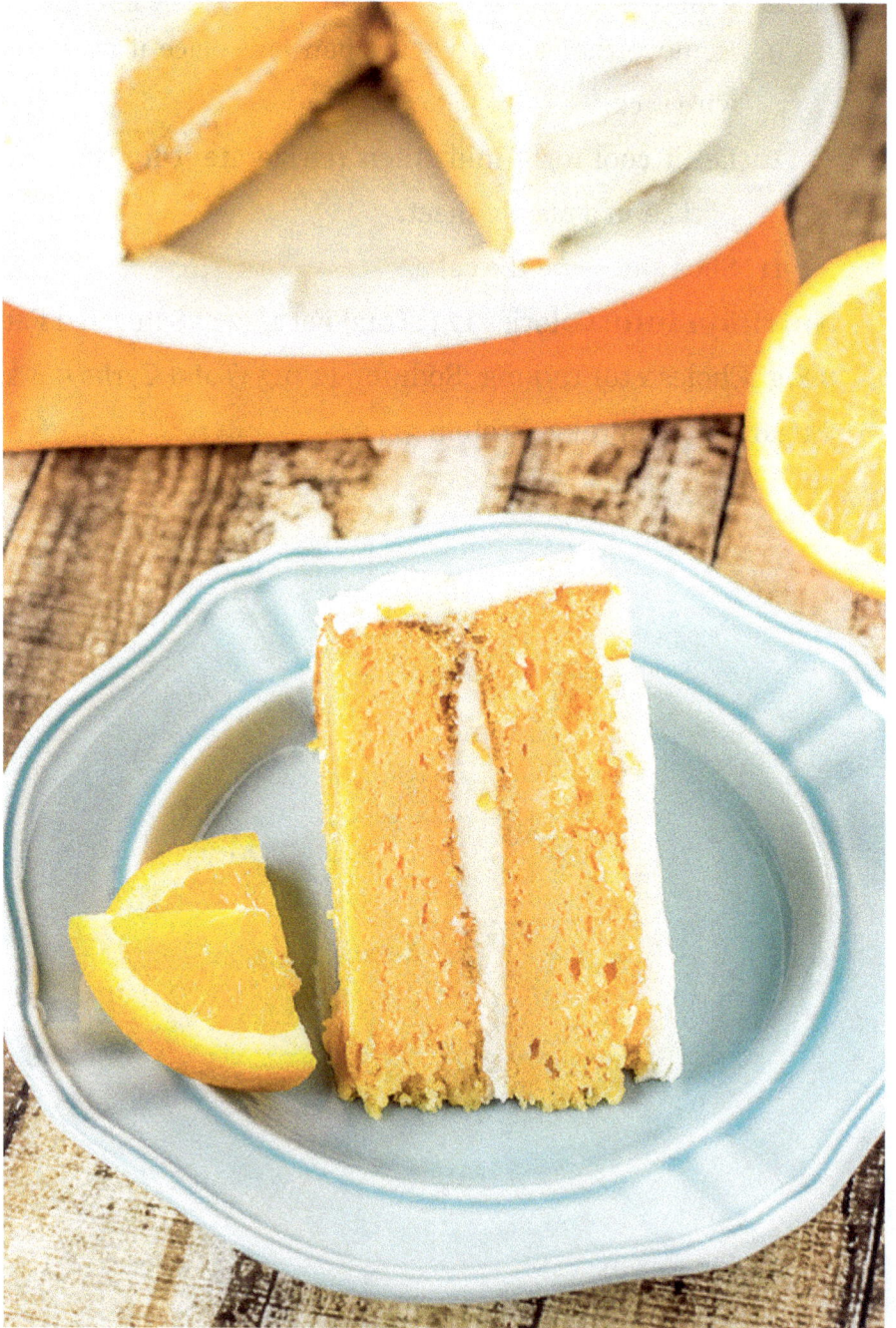

Citrus Cream Cake

Servings: 4

Cooking Time: 60 Minutes

Ingredients:

- Cake
- ¾ teaspoons vanilla essence
- 4 whole eggs
- ¼ cup butter, unsalted softened
- 1 ¼ cups almond flour
- 3/4 cup erythritol
- ¼ teaspoon lemon essence
- ¼ teaspoon salt
- 4 ounces cream cheese
- ¾ teaspoons baking powder
- Cream Frosting
- 1/8 cup erythritol
- 1 ½ tablespoon heavy whipping cream
- ¼ teaspoon vanilla essence

Directions:

1. Adjust the oven at 350 degrees F to preheat.
2. Meanwhile, beat butter with erythritol and cream cheese in a suitable bowl.
3. Stir in eggs, lemon essence and vanilla beat well.
4. Whisk in baking powder, salt, and almond flour.

5. Once the batter is combined well transfer it to a greased baking pan.

6. Bake the cake in preheated oven for minutes at 350 degrees.

7. Beat all the ingredients for the frosting in a suitable bowl.

8. Once done, remove the cake from the pan and place it over the wire rack.

9. Let it cool for 10 mins then spread the cream frosting on its top.

10. Refrigerate the cake for 30 minutes or more.

11. Slice and serve to enjoy.

Nutrition Info: Calories 255 ;Total Fat 23.4 g ;Saturated Fat 11.7 g ;Cholesterol 135 mg ;Sodium 1mg ;Total Carbs 2.5 g ;Sugar 12.5 g ;Fiber 1 g ;Protein 7.9 g

Flourless Chocó Cake

Servings: 8

Cooking Time: 45 Minutes

Ingredients:

- 7 oz unsweetened dark chocolate, chopped
- ¼ cup Swerve
- 4 eggs, separated
- 3.5 oz cream
- 3.5 oz butter, cubed

Directions:

1. Grease 8-inch cake pan with butter and set aside.
2. Add butter and chocolate in microwave safe bowl and microwave until melted. Stir well.
3. Add sweetener and cream and mix well.
4. Add egg yolks one by one and mix until combined.
5. In another bowl, beat egg whites until stiff peaks form.
6. Gently fold egg whites into the chocolate mixture.
7. Pour batter in the prepared cake pan and bake at 325 F 162 C for 45 minutes.
8. Slice and serve.

Nutrition Info: Per Servings: Net Carbs: 5.1g; Calories: 318; Total Fat: 28.2g; Saturated Fat: 17g Protein: 6.6g; Carbs: 8.4g; Fiber: 3.3g; Sugar: 1.2g; Fat 82% Protein 10% Carbs 8%

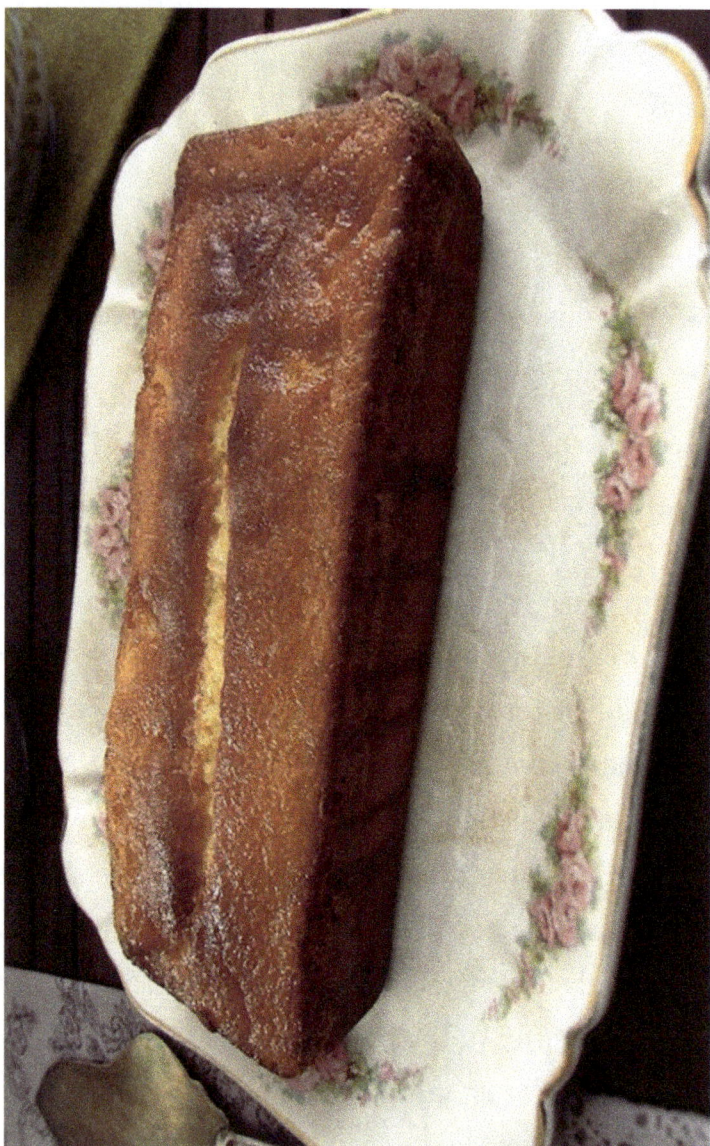

Zesty Lemon Cake

Servings: 8

Cooking Time: 45 Minutes

Ingredients:

- Cake
- 1/2 cup coconut flour
- 5 eggs
- 1/4 cup Swerve
- 1/2 cup butter, melted
- Juice from 1/2 lemon
- 1/2 teaspoon lemon zest
- 1/2 teaspoon xanthan gum
- 1/2 teaspoon salt
- Icing
- 1 cup cream cheese
- 3 tablespoons swerve
- 1 teaspoon vanilla essence
- ½ teaspoon lemon zest

Directions:

1. Whisk egg whites using an electric mixer until it forms stiff peaks.
2. Put everything else in another bowl and mix them well.
3. Once well-combined fold in egg white foam and whisk it gently.

4. Use a spatula to transfer the batter to a 9x5 inch loaf pan, greased with oil.

5. Bake the foamy batter in a preheated oven for 4minutes at 335 degrees F.

6. Meanwhile, prepare the topping by beating icing ingredients in the electric mixer.

7. Place the baked cake on the wire rack and let it cool for 10 minutes.

8. Spread the cream cheese icing over the cake and spread it evenly.

9. Refrigerate for 30 minutes or more.

10. Garnish as desired.

11. Slice and enjoy after a meal.

Nutrition Info: Calories 251 ;Total Fat 24.5 g ;Saturated Fat 14.7 g ;Cholesterol 165 mg ;Sodium 142 mg ;Total Carbs 4.3 g ;Sugar 0.5 g ;Fiber 1 g ;Protein 5.9 g

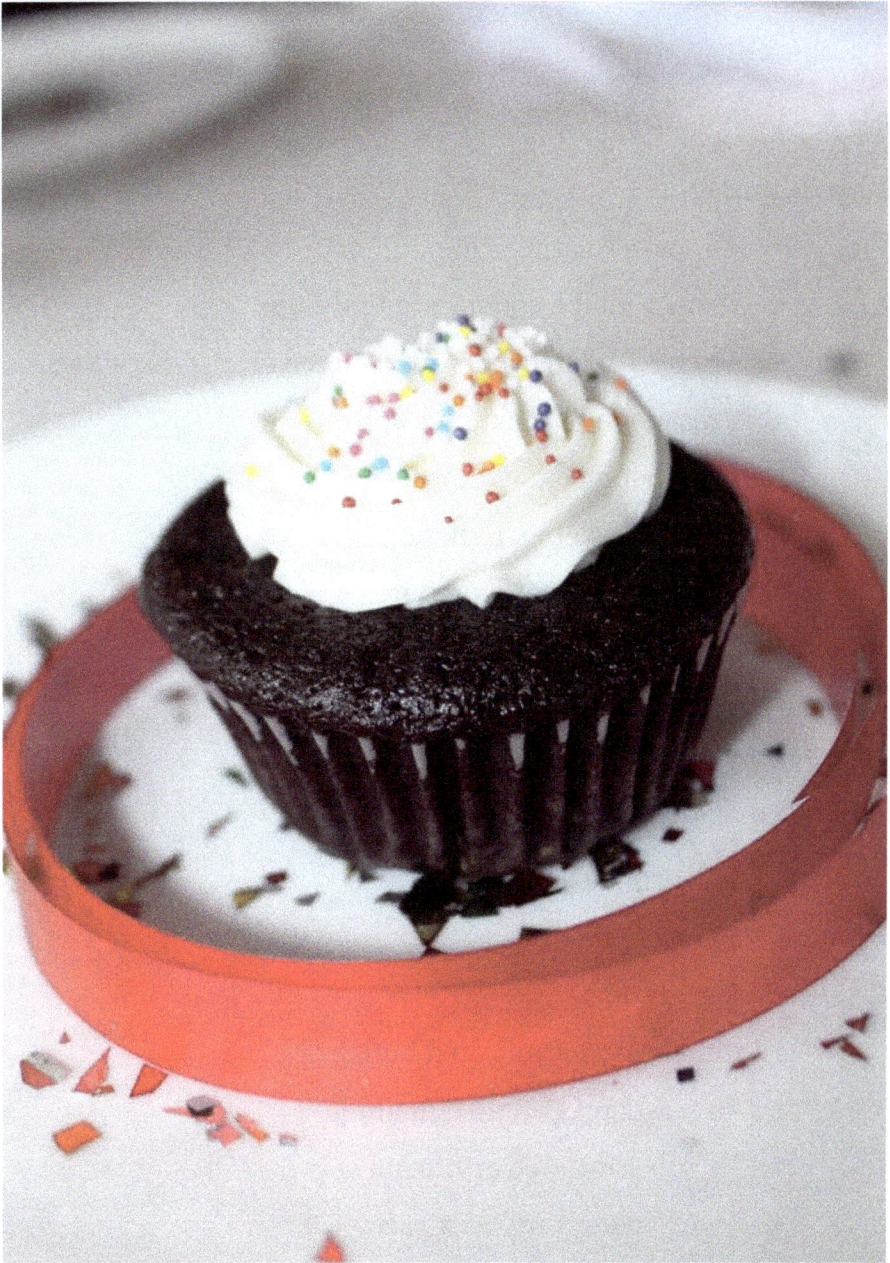

Keto Pumpkin Bundt Cake

Servings: 6

Cooking Time: 45 Minutes

Ingredients:

- For cake (dry ingredients):
- 1 cup + 2 tablespoons almond flour
- ½ cup + 3 tablespoons powdered erythritol or Swerve
- 1 teaspoon pumpkin pie spice
- 1 teaspoon baking powder
- For cake (wet ingredients):
- 4.25 ounces pumpkin puree
- ¼ cup butter or ghee, melted
- 3 large eggs
- 1 teaspoon sugar-free vanilla extract
- ¼ teaspoon salt
- To sprinkle: Optional
- Powdered erythritol
- For glaze:
- 2 tablespoons unsalted butter or ghee
- ½ teaspoon ground cinnamon
- ¼ cup powdered erythritol
- ½ teaspoon vanilla extract

Directions:

1. Add all the dry ingredients into a large mixing bowl.

2. Add the wet ingredients and beat with an electric hand mixer until well incorporated.

3. Spray a small bundt pan with cooking spray.

4. Spoon the batter into the bundt pan.

5. Bake in a preheated oven at 32 F for about 45 minutes. A toothpick when inserted in the center should come out clean when the cake is ready.

6. Cool completely. Invert onto a serving platter.

7. To make the frosting: Add all the ingredients for the glaze into a small pan. Place the pan over low heat. Stir until well combined. Turn off the heat.

8. Spread the glaze over the cake. Sprinkle on some erythritol if desired on top.

9. Cut into slices and serve.

10. Leftovers can be stored in an airtight container in the refrigerator. This can keep for 5 days.

Nutrition Info: Per Servings: Calories: 397.5 kcal, Fat: 28.2 g, Carbohydrates: 7 g, Protein: 7 g

Lemon Poppy Seed Cake

Servings: 16

Cooking Time: 1 Hour And 30 Minutes

Ingredients:

- 3 cups almond flour
- 3 tablespoons poppy seeds
- 2 teaspoons baking powder
- 1/2 teaspoon sea salt
- 1 cup erythritol sweetener
- 2 tablespoons lemon extract, unsweetened
- 2 teaspoons vanilla extract, unsweetened
- 3/4 cup unsalted butter, softened
- 4 eggs
- 3/4 cup sour cream

Directions:

1. Set oven to 350 degrees F and let preheat.
2. Take a Bundt pan, grease with oil and set aside until required.
3. Place butter and sweetener in a bowl and beat with an electric beater until creamy.
4. Then beat in extracts, sour cream, and eggs, one at a time, until smooth.
5. Place flour in another bowl, add poppy seeds, baking powder, and salt and stir well.

6. Stir the flour mixture into butter mixture, ¼ cup at a time, until incorporated.

7. Spoon the batter into prepared Bundt pan and place into the oven to bake for 40 minutes or until top is dark golden brown.

8. Then cover the pan with aluminum foil and continue baking for 20 to 35 minutes or until an inserted toothpick into the cake comes out clean.

9. When done, let bake cool for 15 minutes and then turn it out to cool completely on wire rack.

10. Slice to serve.

Nutrition Info: Calories: 248 Cal, Carbs: 6 g, Fat: 23 g, Protein: 7 g, Fiber: 2 g.

Vanilla Gluten-free Cake

Servings: 12

Cooking Time: 45-50 Minutes

Ingredients:

- For cake:
- ½ cup erythritol
- 4 large eggs
- ½ tablespoon vanilla extract
- 6 tablespoons butter, softened
- ¼ cup unsweetened almond milk
- 1 ½ cups blanched almond flour
- ¾ tablespoon baking powder
- ¼ cup coconut flour
- For cream cheese frosting:
- 16 ounces cream cheese, softened
- 1/3 cup powdered erythritol or more to taste
- 3 tablespoons butter, softened
- ½ teaspoon vanilla extract
- Chopped pecans to garnish (optional)

Directions:

1. Place a round sheet of parchment paper on the bottom of a springform pan of about 6 inches.
2. Add butter and erythritol into a mixing bowl. Beat with an electric hand mixer until creamy.

3. Add eggs, one at a time and beat well each time.

4. Add almond milk and vanilla and beat well.

5. Add the flour and baking powder and beat until well incorporated.

6. Bake in 3 batches to make 3 cakes for a 3-layered cake.

7. Pour 1/3 of the batter into the prepared pan.

8. Bake in a preheated oven at 350° F for about 120 minutes or a toothpick when inserted in the center comes out clean. Remove from the oven and set aside to cool for a while.

9. Remove the cake from the pan and set aside.

10. Repeat steps 7-9 twice more. So in all you will have 3 cakes.

11. To make frosting: Add all the ingredients for the frosting into a mixing bowl.

12. Beat with an electric hand mixer until creamy.

13. Place one cake on a serving platter. Spread 1/3 of the frosting over the cake and the sides as well. Place the 2nd cake over the frosting. Spread 1/3 of the frosting on top and sides as well. Place the 3rd cake and spread remaining frosting over the cake and the sides.

14. Scatter chopped pecans on top if using.

15. Chill for minutes.

16. Slice and serve.

17. Leftovers can be stored in an airtight container in the refrigerator. This can keep for a week

Nutrition Info: Per Servings: Calories: 321.3 kcal, Fat: 17.4 g, Carbohydrates: 5.4 g, Protein: 6 g

Tiramisu Poke Cake

Servings: 6

Cooking Time: 2 – 3 Hours

Ingredients:

- For cake (wet ingredients):
- 3 large eggs
- ¼ cup lukewarm almond milk
- ¼ cup melted ghee or butter
- For cake (dry ingredients):
- 1/3 cup coconut flour
- 1 cup almond flour
- 2 tablespoons whey protein powder or egg white protein powder
- ¼ teaspoon baking soda
- A pinch sea salt or Himalayan pink salt
- 3 tablespoons granulated Swerve or erythritol
- ½ teaspoon cream of tartar or apple cider vinegar
- For coffee-rum custard filling:
- 2 egg yolks
- 6 tablespoons unsweetened almond milk
- ¼ cup strong, brewed coffee
- 1 tablespoon water
- Stevia drops to taste (optional)
- 1 ½ tablespoons granulated Swerve or erythritol

- 1 tablespoon heavy whipping cream
- ½ teaspoon grass-fed gelatin powder
- 2 tablespoons dark rum or ½ teaspoon rum extract
- For mascarpone topping:
- 1 large egg, separated, at room temperature
- 2 tablespoons powdered erythritol or Swerve
- ½ teaspoon vanilla extract
- ½ tablespoon water
- ¼ cup mascarpone, at room temperature
- ½ tablespoon cacao powder

Directions:

1. Place a sheet of firm and strong parchment paper (for example, parchment paper that has foil on one side) on the bottom of the slow cooker. Set on low heat.

2. Add all the wet ingredients into a mixing bowl and whisk well. If you are using apple cider vinegar, add now and whisk well.

3. Add all the dry ingredients into the food processor bowl and process until well combined. If you are using cream of tartar add now and pulse again.

4. Pour the wet ingredients into the food processor and blend until well incorporated and smooth.

5. Transfer into the prepared slow cooker. Cook for 2-3 hours or until set on top.

6. Switch off the cooker and uncover. Let the cake cool in the pot completely.

7. To make coffee rum custard filling: Add egg yolks and erythritol into a bowl and beat until foamy. You can use the whites in another recipe (either dessert, or an egg-white omelet, for example). Set aside.

8. Add cream, milk and coffee into a saucepan. Place the saucepan over medium heat.

9. When it comes to a low boil, turn off the heat. Cool for 4-5 minutes. Add a little of the mixture (1-2 tablespoons) into the bowl of yolks and whisk well. Continue adding this mixture until half of it is added.

10. Pour the yolk mixture into the saucepan with remaining coffee mixture. Place the saucepan over low heat. Stir frequently until the mixture shows 70° F on a cooking thermometer.

11. Whisk together water and gelatin in a bowl and pour into the saucepan. Whisk well. Turn off the heat.

12. Stir in the rum and stevia. Transfer into a glass bowl. Cover the bowl with plastic wrap.

13. Refrigerate for 2 hours.

14. Meanwhile, poke the cake at many places using a wooden skewer or back of a wooden spoon.

15. Spoon the custard into the holes and on top of the cake. Let it cool for 2 hours.

16. To make mascarpone topping: Add egg yolk into a heatproof bowl. Add water and beat until frothy. Add vanilla extract and erythritol and whisk until light yellow in color.

17. Place the heatproof bowl in a double boiler. Stir continuously until the mixture begins to thicken (about 6-8 minutes)

18. Turn off the heat and remove the bowl from the double boiler. Stir constantly until it cools.

19. Add mascarpone cheese and fold gently.

20. Add a pinch of salt to the egg white and whip until stiff peaks are formed.

21. Add whites into the bowl of yolk and fold gently.

22. Spread this mixture over the cake.

23. Dust with cocoa powder. Remove the cake from the slow cooker along with the parchment paper and place in the refrigerator. Chill for 3-4 hours.

24. Cut into 6-7 pieces and serve.

25. Leftovers can be stored in an airtight container in the refrigerator. The cake can keep for a week.

Nutrition Info: Per Servings: Calories:359 kcal, Fat: 30.2 g, Carbohydrates: 8.7 g, Protein: 9.3 g

Coconut Cake

Servings: 8

Cooking Time: 20 Minutes

Ingredients:

- 5 eggs, separated
- ½ tsp baking powder
- ½ tsp vanilla
- ½ cup butter softened
- ½ cup erythritol
- ¼ cup unsweetened coconut milk
- ½ cup coconut flour
- Pinch of salt

Directions:

1. Preheat the oven to 400 F 200 C.
2. Grease cake pan with butter and set aside.
3. In a bowl, beat sweetener and butter until combined.
4. Add egg yolks, coconut milk, and vanilla and mix well.
5. Add baking powder, coconut flour, and salt and stir well.
6. In another bowl, beat egg whites until stiff peak forms.
7. Gently fold egg whites into the cake mixture.
8. Pour batter in a prepared cake pan and bake in preheated oven for 20 minutes.
9. Slice and serve.

Nutrition Info: Per Servings: Net Carbs: 0.8g; Calories: 163 Total Fat: 16.2g; Saturated Fat: 9.9g Protein: 3.9g; Carbs: 1.3g; Fiber: 0.5g; Sugar: 0.6g; Fat 89% Protein 9% Carbs 2%

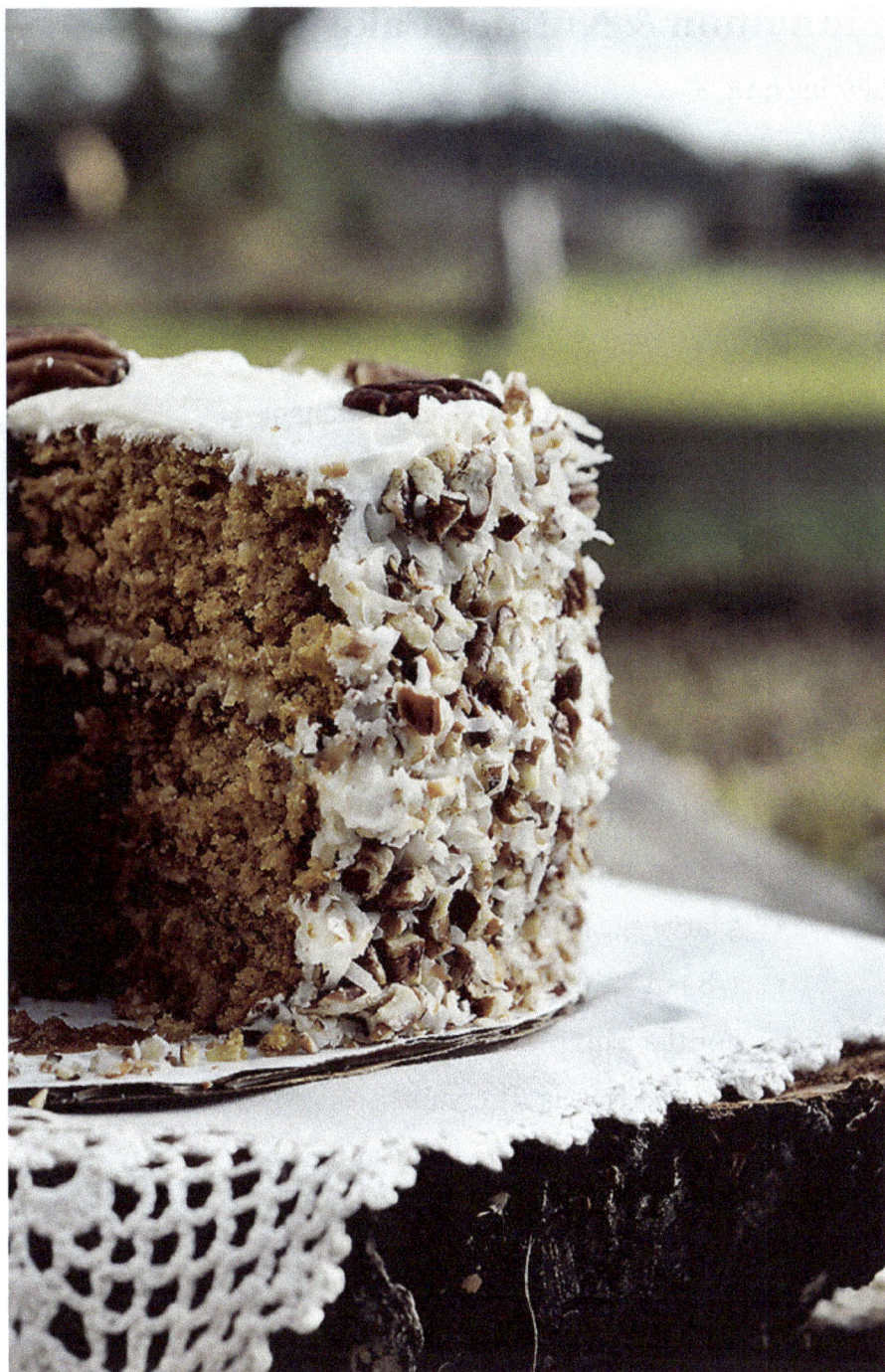

Cinnamon & Nutmeg Cake

Servings: 14

Cooking Time: 1 Hour 55 Minutes

Ingredients:

- For the cake:
- 1 1/2 cups almond flour
- 5 oz. butter, unsalted and softened
- 1 tsp. ground cinnamon
- 3/4 cup sweetener, granulated
- 1 tsp. baking powder, gluten-free
- 2 tbsp. coconut flour
- 1/2 tsp. ground ginger
- 5 oz. cream cheese, softened
- 1/4 tsp. ground cloves
- 1/2 tsp. ground nutmeg
- 5 large eggs
- 1/8 tsp. salt
- For the icing:
- 2/3 cup Natvia icing mix
- 4 oz. butter, unsalted and softened
- 2 tbsp. heavy whipping cream
- 4 oz. cream cheese, softened
- 1 tsp. ground cinnamon

Directions:

1. Cake:
2. Set the temperature of the stove to 350° Fahrenheit. Use butter to liberally grease an 8-inch cake pan and place baking paper to cover the base of the cake pan.In a big dish, blend the cream cheese and baking powder using an electrical beater.
3. Add the butter and sweetener until combined. Then sprinkle the cinnamon, cloves, nutmeg, and salt into the mixture.
4. Combine the almond flour, coconut flour, and eggs making sure there are no lumps present. Use a scraper on the dish and thoroughly mix.
5. Distribute the cake batter in the prepared pan and heat in the stove for 30 − 40 minutes. Ensure it is baked all the way through by poking a toothpick into the middle.
6. Remove the pan and place on the cake platter. Set to the side.
7. Frosting:
8. In a regular dish, blend cream cheese until the mixture is creamy.
9. Combine the butter and mix thoroughly.
10. Add the Natvia icing mix one spoonful at a time to ensure it gets completely mixed. Then combine the heavy whipping cream and cinnamon, continuing to stir the frosting until smooth.

11. Frost the middle first and then complete the frosting process after the cake has completely cooled.

12. Tricks and Tips:

13. You can store this cake in the freezer for up to 3 months. Make sure it is wrapped tightly with plastic wrap or a freezer ziplock bag.

Nutrition Info: 7 grams ;Net Carbs: 3 grams ;Fat: 24 grams ;Calories: 374

Double Layer Cream Cake

Servings: 8

Cooking Time: 25 Minutes

Ingredients:

- First Layer
- 3 tablespoons coconut flour
- 1/4 cup erythritol, powdered
- 1 teaspoon baking powder
- 1 tablespoon gelatine
- 8 tablespoons butter
- 1/2 teaspoon vanilla essence
- 2 large eggs,
- Second Layer
- 8 tablespoons butter,
- 8 oz. cream cheese,
- 1/2 teaspoon vanilla essence
- Liquid stevia, to taste
- 2 large eggs,

Directions:

1. Let your oven preheat at 350 degrees F.
2. Take an 8-inch springform pan and butter it to grease well.
3. First layer
4. Beat vanilla and butter in all the eggs in a mixer.

5. Stir in gelatine, baking powder, flour, and gelatine.

6. Mix well until everything is well incorporated. Set this mixture aside.

7. Second Layer

8. Beat the butter with cream cheese separately in an electric mixer.

9. Add stevia and vanilla essence for flavor. Then whisk in eggs.

10. Beat everything until the mixture is smooth.

11. Assembly:

12. First spread the first layer in the greased baking pan.

13. Then top this layer with batter from the second layer evenly.

14. Bake the cake for 25 minutes in the preheated oven.

15. Once done, remove the cake from the oven and allow it to cool on wire rack,

16. Refrigerate for 2 hours in a wrapped plastic sheet.

17. Slice and serve.

Nutrition Info: Calories 336 ;Total Fat 34.5 g ;Saturated Fat 21.4 g ;Cholesterol 139 mg ;Sodium 267 mg ;Total Carbs 9.1 g ;Sugar 0.2 g ;Fiber 1.1 g ;Protein 5.1 g

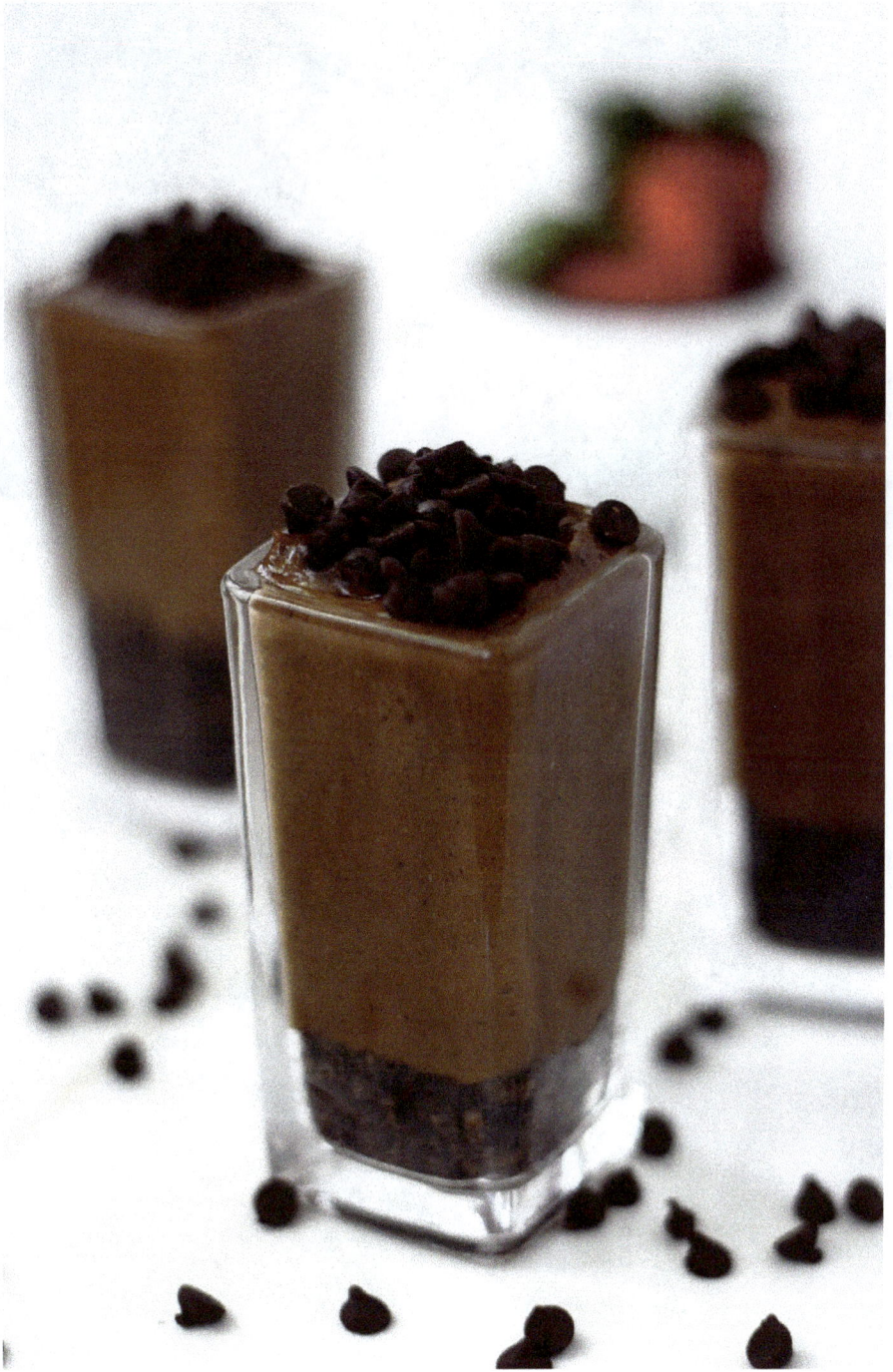

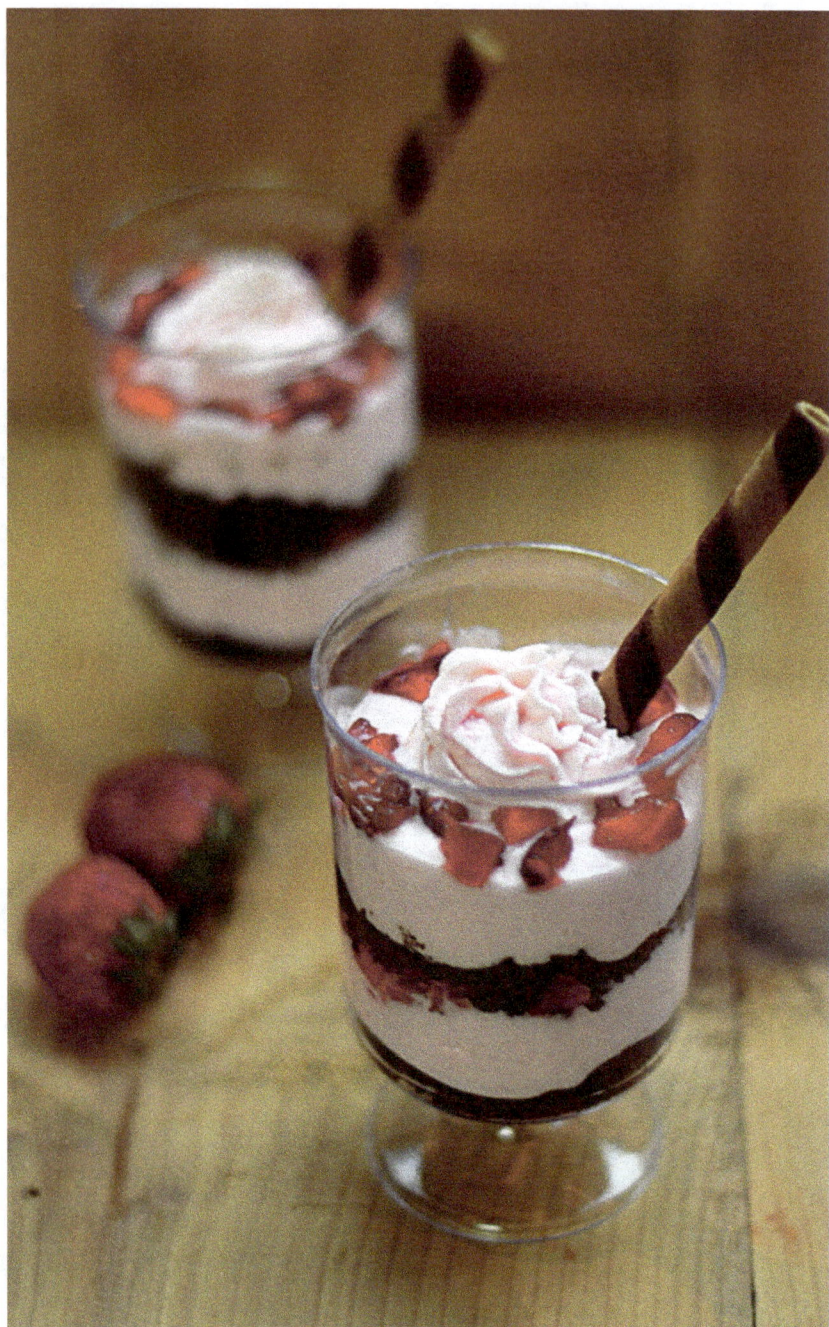